TABLE OF CONTENTS

Success Lies Ahead! 4

How To Use This Book 4

Welcome to Hospital Nursing 5

Understanding the Hospital Ecosystem 6

Structure of a Hospital: Departments and Units... 6

Communication Skills with Patients, Families, and Healthcare Team 14

Escalation Hierarchy 16

How do I figure out what I need to do? 16

What does a 12-hour shift look like? 17

Assessment & Management of Patient Conditions By Body System 21

Circulatory System 21

Digestive System 24

Endocrine-These conditions often involve hormonal imbalances that affect various body systems 29

Immune System 34

Integumentary System... 39

Muscular System... 43

Nervous System 47

Reproductive System 51

Respiratory System 55

Urinary System 60

Navigating Patient Care 65

Ethical Considerations in Patient Care 65

Hospital Nursing Procedures and Protocols 69

Infection Control and Prevention Measures 69

Documentation and Charting Standards 72

Coping with Challenges in Hospital Nursing 74

Handling Stress and Burnout 74

Dealing with Critical Situations and Emergencies 74

Conclusion 76

Recap of Essential Points Covered 76

Encouragement for Aspiring and Current Nurses 76

Final Thoughts and Resources for Further Learning 77

Special Formulas 79

Success Lies Ahead!

The goal of nursing school is to prepare you to pass the NCLEX. It doesn't prepare you to care for patients and hit the ground running. In fact, we are left with so many unanswered questions and become overwhelmed with anxiety because we no longer have the safety net that our classroom provided. This book is going to bridge that gap between classroom and bedside. When I got my first hospital job me and every single new grad that I knew were so lost, frustrated, and overwhelmed during our internship. It took me months to be confident caring for patients on my own. It took others longer, and some quit before they could even complete the internship. I remember asking my manager if there was a guide from the hospital to help support us new nurses but it didn't exist, until now.

This book is going to give you answers to questions you didn't even know you had and give you the information that you need to build your confidence in the acute care setting as a bedside nurse. Not only will this book prepare you for what to expect during your shift, it will help guide you when providing care to your patients so that you can begin connecting the dots on your own, sooner rather than later. This book is a must read to any new grad, experienced nurse, or nurse transitioning to the acute care setting.

How To Use This Book

This book is very concise and straight to the point. I know your time is limited so I wanted the information to be accessible and easy to flip through. Here you will find some of the most common situations found in the acute care hospital setting with reasoning to help put pieces of the puzzle together. **Disclaimer,** all hospitals run slightly differently than others, yet they also all have the same functional principles. By no means is this book meant to replace your critical thinking skills or should it be used in an emergency. This is a great guide to review in your leisure so that you can properly retain this information, connect the dots, then apply it to your patient centered care. Let's get in to it!

Welcome to Hospital Nursing

Nurses make up the majority of staff in the hospital setting. We are responsible for being the doctor's eyes and ears when they are not present to assess patients. Nurses wear many hats, but our utmost responsibility is to be our patient's advocate. Every time you see your patient you are assessing them. Nursing in a hospital setting is an entire new world by itself and can be quite difficult to navigate without the proper guidance. This book will provide concise information for prioritization, protocols, necessary assessments based on patient illness and body systems and critical thinking exercises.

You Got This! *Bridging the Gap between Bedside Nursing* will guide you and build upon the foundation of your nursing care.

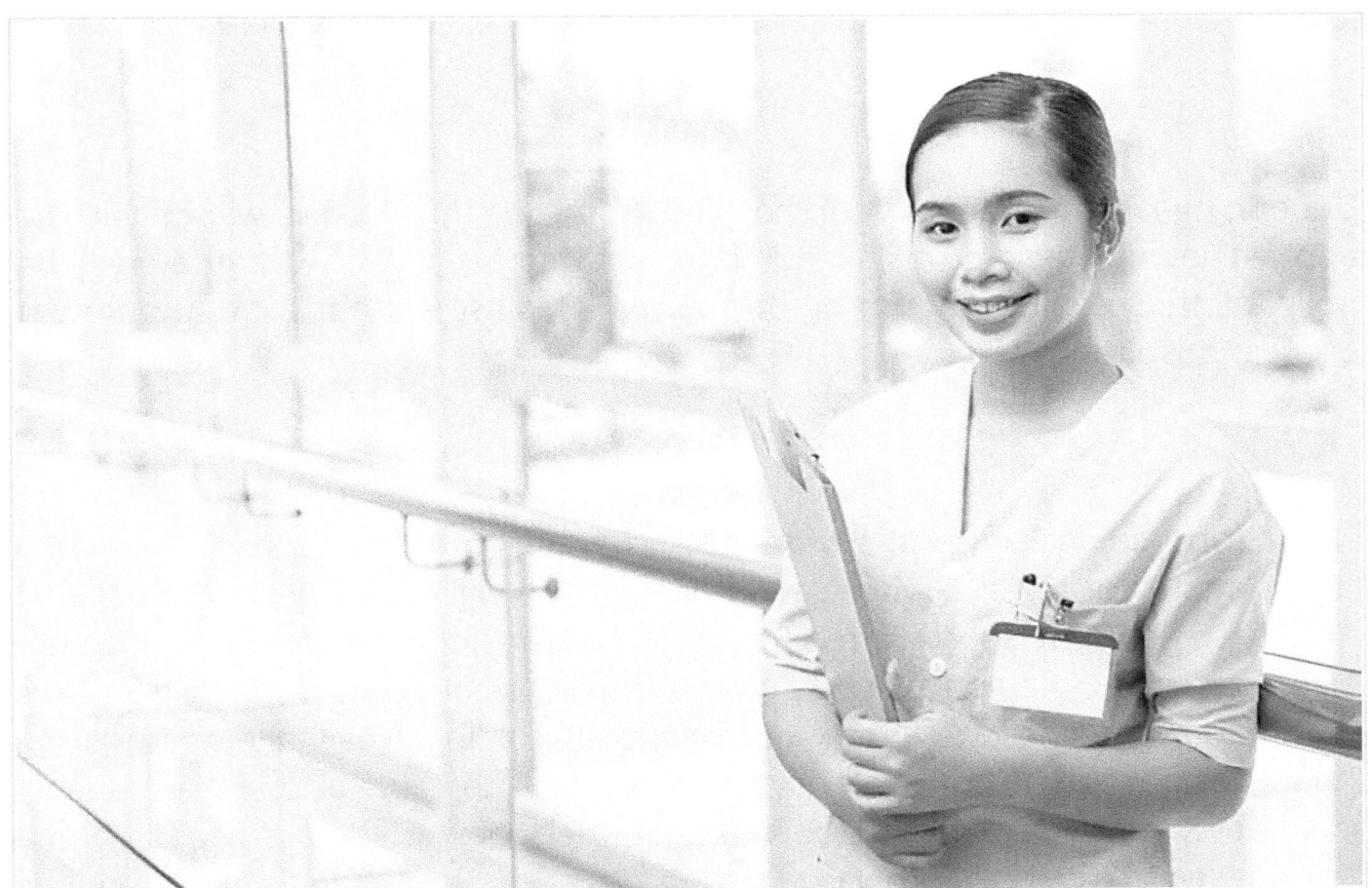

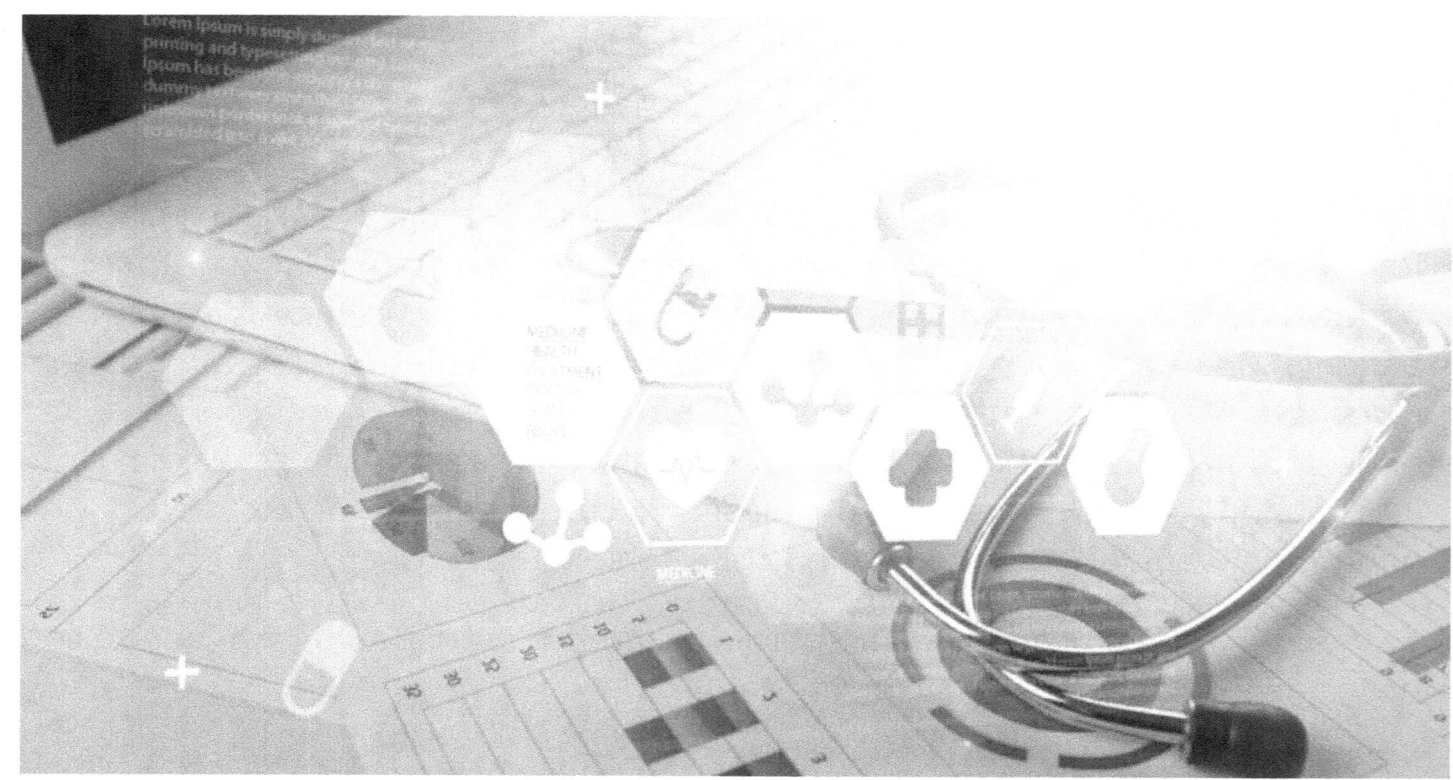

Understanding the Hospital Ecosystem

Depending on the size of your hospital, some of these units will or will not apply. They may also go by slightly different names. If you work in a specialty hospital, those units may not be on this list. This list is the meat and potatoes of most hospital systems.

Structure of a Hospital: Departments and Units

- **Emergency Room/ER Holds-** This is where most patients initiate care. Patients of all ages will be seen here. Some will be seen, prescribed a Rx then go home shortly after. Some will be transferred to specialty hospitals (pediatrics, trauma centers, stroke hospitals...etc.). Those being admitted and are medically stable will go to the ER holding area while waiting for a room on a unit. You will have a mixture of unstable and stable patients here. Patients are stabilized in the ER, then they will be assigned to a unit based off their acuity level.

- **Clinical Decision Unit (CDU)-** This may also be called the observation unit. Patients here are medically stable and are thought to only need observation for 24-48 hrs. Depending on your state, nurses may have 5-6 patients, depending on their acuity level.

- **Medical/Surgical-** Patients are sent here who are medically stable. Depending on your state, nurses can have anywhere between 5-6 patients. Depending on acuity level.

- **Progressive Care Unit (PCU)/Telemetry-** Patients on this unit need closer monitoring. Patients requiring IV drips with titrating, hourly vitals, cardiac monitoring, stroke patients, cardiac procedures, frequent neuro checks, increased respiratory support to name a few will be cared for here. Nurses ideally will have 3-4 patients. Depending on acuity level.

- **Intensive Care Unit (ICU)-** Patients here are not medically stable and require even closer observation. This is the most advanced level of care in the hospital. Nurses may have 1-3 patients at a time. Depending on acuity level.

- **Dialysis-** Small unit within hospital. May only have 5-6 beds, depending on the size of the hospital. The highest ratio I've seen is 1:8, but I have seen that some nurses can have up to 20 patients. That is usually at an outpatient Dialysis center.

- **Post Anesthesia Care Unit (PACU)-** Patients go here after surgery to recover from anesthesia. They are monitored for 1-3 hours depending on the type of surgery, medical history, and patient response. Nurses may have 1-2 patients at a time. Depending on acuity level.

- **OrthoSurgical/Trauma-** Sometimes these units are separate. Ortho unit focuses on patients that have bone fractures. Most fractures are caused by a traumatic event so you may also see trauma patients as well. Mvc's, injuries from falls, injuries at work make up some of the patient population.

- **Rehabilitation-** This is where patients go to receive therapy to aid their recovery. Usually Speech therapy, occupational therapy, and physical therapy are involved. Patients recovering from broken bones or debilitating illnesses may decide they need additional help before they return home. Nurses may have 5-6 patients, depending on acuity

- **Labor & Delivery/Postpartum-** This is where our babies are born. Nurses may have 1:2 patient in L&D, 1:3 postpartum, and 1:6 in the well-baby nursery

- **Neonatal Intensive Care Unit-** Our preemies and medically unstable newborns will go here. Nurse ratio may be 1:2.

- **Introduction to Hospital Protocols and Policies-** Always follow your hospital policies and protocols. If you float between multiple hospitals, be sure to familiarize yourself with each of the hospitals policies. I've seen hospitals that require phlebotomy to start IV's to help free up nurses. I've also seen hospitals without phlebotomist tech that require nurses to do all lab draws.

- **Interdisciplinary Collaboration:** Working with Doctors, Technicians, and Support Staff.

- **Hospitalist-** General physician that oversees the care of patients. There should be one assigned to each patient. The hospitalist assists in making sure all members of the care team are communicating accordingly and on the same page. Reach out to them for basic orders (pain meds, diet, med reconciliation..etc.). ***Under NO circumstances should any therapies, medications may be pursued without a MD order***.

- **Specialist-** Specialty physician that focuses on care of a particular body system. E.g., endocrinologist, cardiologist, hematologist...etc. Reach out to them for orders that correspond with their specialty. For example, if you need an order for a kidney patient to have IV fluids, the best MD to ask will be the nephrologist, then the hospitalist.

- **Trauma Surgeons**- Group of doctors that specialize in traumatic injuries that involve surgery. Some of these patients may suffer from ground level falls, mvc's, gallbladder, and appendix issues.

- **Speech Therapist**- Speech therapists play a crucial role in assessing and treating communication and swallowing disorders in patients of all ages. They work with patients who have suffered from conditions such as strokes, traumatic brain injuries, or neurological disorders, helping them regain speech and language skills. Additionally, speech therapists provide swallowing evaluations and therapy to ensure safe swallowing function, collaborating closely with other healthcare professionals to optimize patient outcomes and quality of life. Reach out to them if your patient has dysphagia and needs evaluations before starting a diet.

- **Physical Therapist**- Physical therapists focus on restoring mobility, strength, and function in patients recovering from injury, surgery, or illness. They conduct comprehensive assessments to determine the patient's physical limitations and develop personalized treatment plans, which may include therapeutic exercises, manual therapy techniques, and mobility training. Physical therapists also educate patients and caregivers on proper body mechanics and exercise regimens to facilitate recovery and prevent future injuries. Additionally, they collaborate with other healthcare team members to ensure coordinated care and optimal patient outcomes

- **Occupational Therapist-** Occupational therapists assist patients in regaining independence in activities of daily living (ADLs) and improving functional abilities necessary for returning home or to a community setting. They assess the patient's physical, cognitive, and emotional status to develop individualized treatment plans aimed at promoting independence in self-care, work, and leisure activities. Occupational therapists also provide adaptive equipment recommendations and environmental modifications to facilitate safe and efficient performance of daily tasks, collaborating with other healthcare professionals to optimize patient outcomes and transitions to home or community settings.

- **Charge Nurse/Supervisor-** The charge nurse assumes a leadership role responsible for overseeing a specific unit or shift. They coordinate patient care activities, delegate tasks to nursing staff, and ensure that policies and procedures are followed. Additionally, charge nurses serve as a resource for nursing staff, address any patient care concerns or emergencies that arise, and facilitate communication between healthcare team members to promote efficient and effective patient care delivery.

- **House Supervisor-** House supervisor, often referred to as a nursing supervisor, plays a pivotal role in overseeing the daily operations of patient care units. They manage staffing levels, coordinate patient admissions and discharges, and address any issues or concerns that arise during their shift. House supervisors also serve as a resource for nursing staff, provide support in emergencies, and ensure that hospital policies and procedures are followed to maintain quality patient care and safety throughout the facility.

- **Director/Clinical Manager-** a Clinical Manager oversees the daily operations of a specific clinical department or unit, such as nursing, respiratory therapy, or radiology. They are responsible for staffing, scheduling, and ensuring adequate resources to meet patient care needs while adhering to budgetary constraints. Clinical Managers also play a key role in developing and implementing policies and procedures to maintain high-quality patient care, foster staff development, and ensure compliance with regulatory standards. Additionally, they serve as liaisons between frontline staff, hospital administration, and other healthcare professionals to promote effective communication and teamwork.

- **CNO/Assoc CNO-** The Chief Nursing Officer (CNO) in a hospital setting is responsible for overseeing all nursing operations and ensuring the delivery of high-quality patient care. They collaborate with other members of the executive team to develop and implement strategic initiatives aimed at improving nursing practices, patient outcomes, and organizational efficiency. Additionally, the CNO plays a key role in fostering a positive work environment for nursing staff, promoting professional development, and maintaining compliance with regulatory standards and best practices in healthcare.

- **Respiratory Nurses-** Respiratory nurses plays a vital role in caring for patients with acute and chronic respiratory conditions. They assess patients' respiratory status, administer treatments such as oxygen therapy, chest physiotherapy, and nebulization, and monitor respiratory equipment. Respiratory nurses also educate patients and their families on respiratory care techniques, medication administration, and disease management to promote optimal lung function and improve overall respiratory health. Additionally, they collaborate with other healthcare professionals to develop and implement comprehensive care plans tailored to each patient's needs.

- **Dialysis Nurses-** Dialysis nurses plays a vital role in providing specialized care to patients undergoing dialysis treatment for kidney failure. They are responsible for assessing patients before, during, and after dialysis sessions, monitoring vital signs, and ensuring the safety and comfort of patients throughout the procedure. Dialysis nurses also educate patients and their families on kidney disease management, dietary restrictions, and medication adherence, while collaborating closely with nephrologists and other healthcare professionals to optimize patient outcomes and manage complications associated with kidney failure.

- **Patient Care Techs (PCT/CNA)-** a patient care technician (PCT) provides direct care and support to patients under the supervision of registered nurses or other healthcare professionals. Their responsibilities typically include assisting patients with activities of daily living such as bathing, dressing, and feeding, taking vital signs, and transporting patients. Patient care technicians also play a vital role in maintaining a clean and safe environment for patients, assisting with medical procedures, and documenting patient information accurately.

- **Telemetry Techs-** Telemetry technician's plays a vital role in monitoring patients' cardiac activity using specialized equipment such as telemetry monitors. Telemetry techs promptly identify and report any abnormalities in heart rhythms, allowing for timely intervention and treatment by healthcare providers. Additionally, they may assist with troubleshooting technical issues related to telemetry monitoring systems to ensure continuous and reliable monitoring of patients' cardiac status.

- **EKG Techs**- EKG (electrocardiogram) technicians are responsible for performing non-invasive tests to record the electrical activity of a patient's heart. They apply electrodes to the patient's chest, limbs, and sometimes the neck area to capture the heart's electrical impulses accurately. EKG technicians also ensure the quality of the recorded data, troubleshoot any technical issues during testing, and communicate findings to healthcare providers for interpretation and diagnosis.

- **Radiology**- Radiologists are specialized physicians responsible for interpreting medical images such as X-rays, CT scans, MRIs, and ultrasounds. They play a critical role in diagnosing diseases, injuries, and conditions by analyzing and providing detailed reports on imaging findings. Radiologists work closely with other healthcare providers to guide treatment decisions, monitor disease progression, and ensure the accuracy and quality of diagnostic imaging studies for optimal patient care.

- **Nuclear Medicine (NM)**- Nuclear medicine utilizes radioactive materials to diagnose and treat various medical conditions. Nuclear medicine procedures involve administering small amounts of radioactive substances to patients, which are then detected by specialized imaging equipment to provide detailed images of internal organs and tissues. These images help physicians diagnose diseases such as cancer, heart conditions, and neurological disorders, as well as monitor treatment effectiveness. Additionally, nuclear medicine techniques are used in therapeutic procedures, such as targeted radiation therapy for certain cancers, to precisely deliver treatment to diseased tissues while minimizing damage to surrounding healthy cells.

- **Case Management**- Case management involves coordinating and facilitating the care of patients throughout their healthcare journey. Case managers assess patients' needs, develop individualized care plans, and advocate for appropriate services and resources. They collaborate with healthcare providers, patients, and families to ensure continuity of care, streamline communication, and promote efficient utilization of healthcare resources. Case managers also address discharge planning, transition to post-hospital care settings, and facilitate access to community resources for ongoing support.

- **Dietician-** Dietitians play a crucial role in assessing patients' nutritional needs and developing personalized dietary plans to support their overall health and recovery. They collaborate with healthcare teams to address malnutrition, obesity, and other nutrition-related conditions by providing evidence-based nutrition counseling and education. Dietitians also monitor patients' dietary intake, evaluate the effectiveness of dietary interventions, and make adjustments as needed to optimize nutritional status and promote healing. Additionally, they may contribute to discharge planning by providing recommendations for continued nutrition care post-hospitalization.

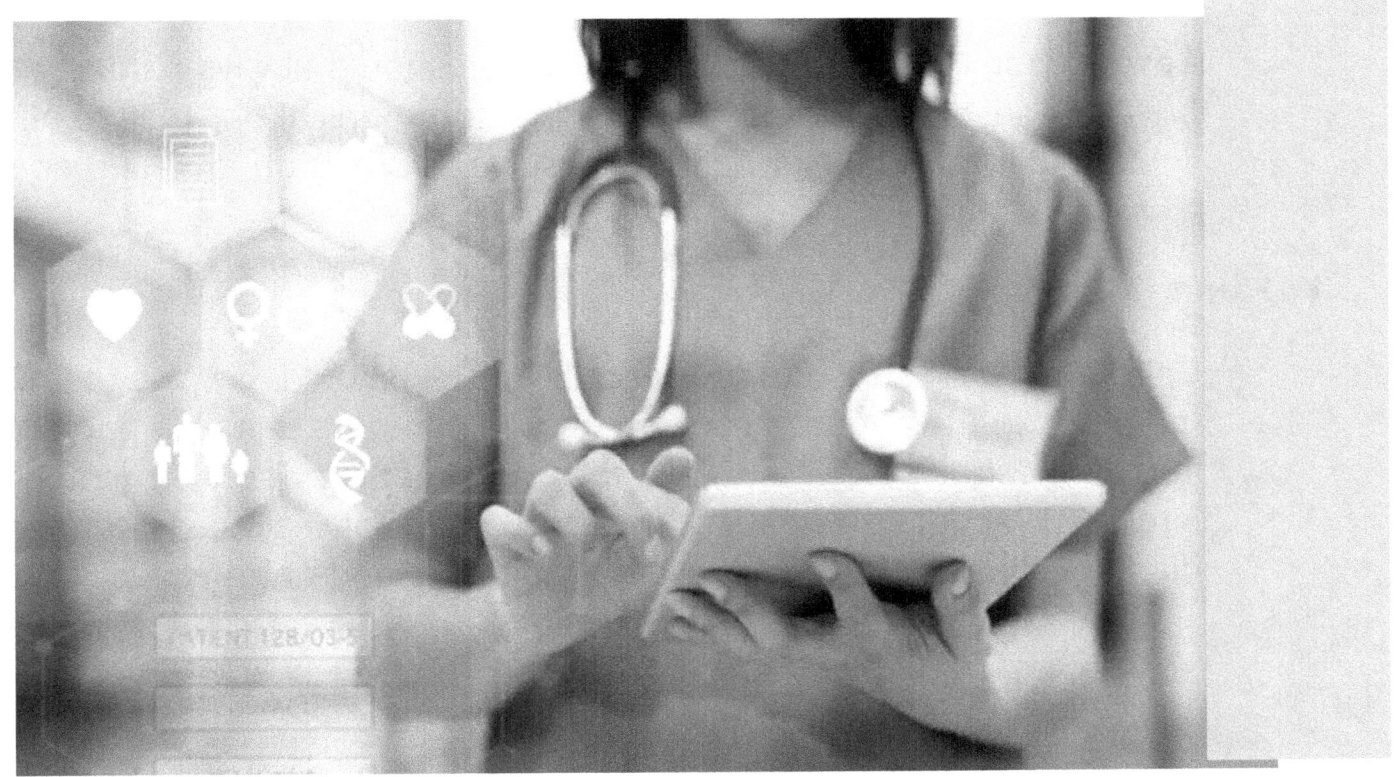

Communication Skills with Patients, Families, and Healthcare Team

- **Patients:**

    - **Clear and Compassionate Communication**: Nurses are expected to communicate with patients in a clear, understandable manner, using language appropriate to the patient's level of comprehension. Compassion and empathy are crucial components of patient communication, as nurses should strive to make patients feel heard, valued, and supported.

    - **Active Listening:** Nurses should actively listen to patients, allowing them to express their concerns, preferences, and needs. This helps build trust and fosters a therapeutic relationship between the nurse and the patient.

    - **Providing Information:** Nurses are responsible for providing patients with information about their health condition, treatment options, and care plan. This empowers patients to make informed decisions about their care and promotes patient autonomy.

    - **Respect for Privacy and Dignity:** Nurses should always respect the privacy and dignity of patients during communication, maintaining confidentiality and ensuring that sensitive information is discussed in a private setting.

- **Family Members:**

    - **Collaboration and Partnership:** Nurses should involve family members in the patient's care, recognizing them as valuable partners in the healthcare team. This involves keeping family members informed about the patient's condition, involving them in care planning discussions, and soliciting their input and preferences.

- - **Support and Empathy:** Family members often experience stress and anxiety when a loved one is hospitalized. Nurses should offer emotional support, empathy, and reassurance to family members, addressing their concerns and answering their questions to the best of their ability.

  - **Setting Realistic Expectations:** If the patient consents to sharing health information- Nurses should communicate openly and honestly with family members about the patient's condition, prognosis, and expected outcomes. Setting realistic expectations helps alleviate uncertainty and facilitates coping and decision-making.

- **Healthcare Team:**

  - **Interdisciplinary Collaboration:** Nurses collaborate with other members of the healthcare team, including physicians, therapists, social workers, and ancillary staff, to ensure coordinated and comprehensive patient care. Effective communication among team members is essential for achieving optimal patient outcomes.

  - **Clear and Concise Reporting:** Nurses provide clear and concise verbal and written reports to other healthcare team members, including relevant patient information, assessments, interventions, and changes in status. This facilitates continuity of care and ensures that all team members are informed and up-to-date.

  - **Advocacy:** Nurses advocate for their patients within the healthcare team, ensuring that their needs and preferences are considered and addressed. Effective communication is key to advocating for patients' rights, safety, and well-being.

Overall, effective communication is fundamental to nursing practice in a hospital setting, fostering therapeutic relationships, promoting patient-centered care, and facilitating collaboration among healthcare team members.

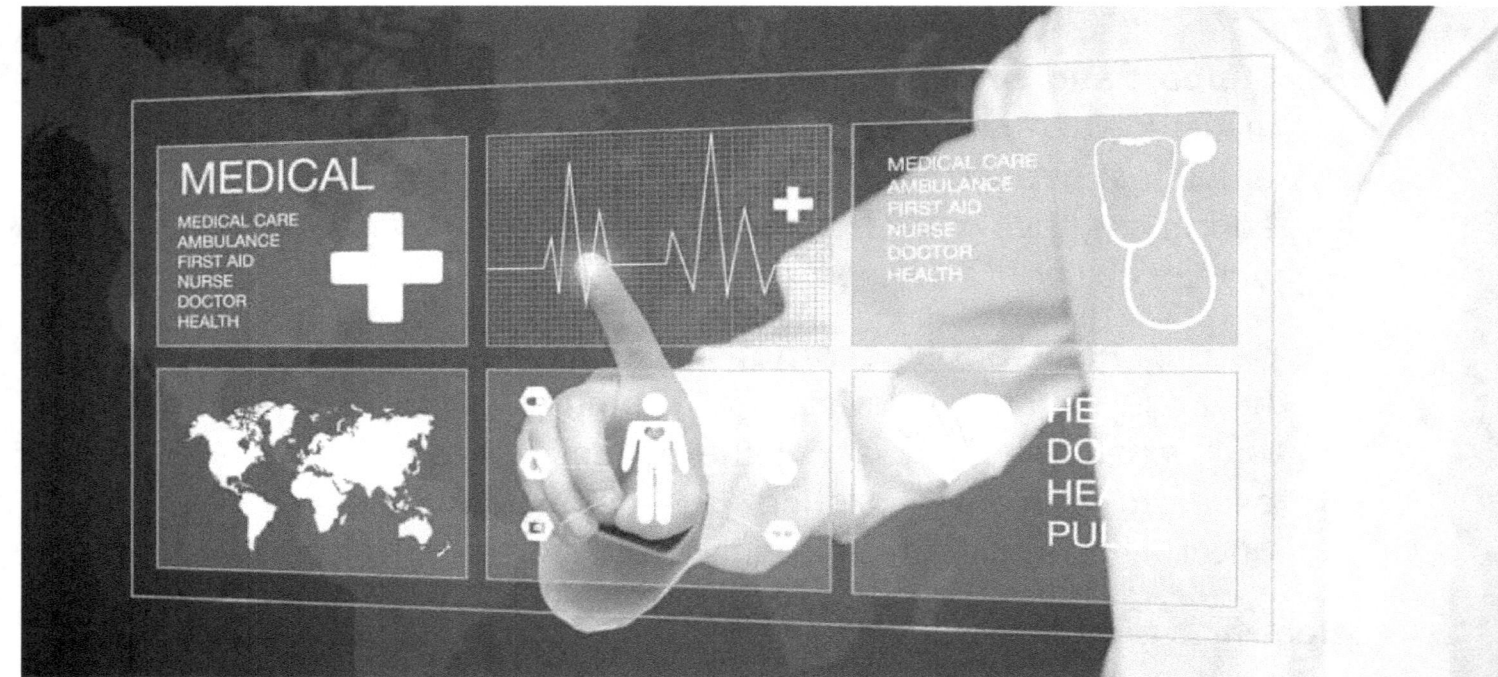

Escalation Hierarchy

How Do I figure out what I need to do?

- **Problem Solving:** You are the Nurse, You must find a resolution of defer to someone who can. Most problems you can handle on your own and with the support of staff.

- When in doubt ask a fellow nurse. If unresolved, ask Charge next. If Charge doesn't resolve you may reach out to House Supervisor.

- Most problems need to be referred to the appropriate department. Having an issue with labs? Contact Lab. Having an issue with medications not scanning? Contact Pharmacy. Why hasn't my patient been taken down to X-Ray, contact imaging...etc

- Call MD to notify him/her of changes in your patient. Most MD's have a NP that is on call for them. Always try to call NP first instead of MD. Certain providers may prefer a text instead of a call. If you have texted and there hasn't been a response you must call. Anything emergent must be a call.

- If your patient is in a crisis and needs immediate intervention call a Code (Rapid Response, Stroke, Blue, Behavioral) then call the MD if appropriate. Stay with your patient.

What does a 12-hour shift look like?

A typical 12-hour shift for a nurse in an acute care setting is fast-paced and involves a wide range of responsibilities. Here's an overview of what the day might look like:

Shift Start: Handoff and Preparation (6:30 AM - 7:00 AM)

- **Pre-Shift Preparation:**
  - Arrive at the hospital, clock in, and attend the shift briefing or huddle.
  - Receive patient assignments from the outgoing shift, including a detailed handoff report using SBAR (Situation, Background, Assessment, Recommendation).

- **Chart Review:**
  - Review patient charts, medical histories, current medications, lab results, and any physician orders.
  - Prioritize patient care based on acuity and needs.

Morning Rounds and Assessments (7:00 AM - 10:00 AM)

- **Patient Assessment:**
  - Conduct head-to-toe assessments on each patient, checking vital signs, reviewing any overnight changes, and assessing pain levels, wounds, or surgical sites.
  - Document findings in the electronic health record (EHR).

- **Medication Administration:**
  - Administer morning medications, including IVs, oral medications, and any scheduled treatments.

- Educate patients on new medications or treatments, addressing any concerns.

- **Rounds with Physicians:**

    - Participate in interdisciplinary rounds with the healthcare team, providing input on patient care and updates on the patient's condition.

    - Update care plans based on new orders or changes discussed during rounds.

Mid-Morning: Patient Care and Procedures (10:00 AM - 12:00 PM)

- **Implement Care Plans:**

    - Carry out care plans, which may include wound care, administering blood transfusions, assisting with diagnostic tests (e.g., EKGs, X-rays), and preparing patients for surgery or procedures.

    - Collaborate with physical therapists, dietitians, or other specialists involved in patient care.

- **Patient Education:**

    - Provide education on disease processes, discharge planning, or post-operative care.

Lunch and Breaks (12:00 PM - 1:00 PM) If you're lucky!

- **Take a Break:**

    - Depending on staffing and patient needs, take a lunch break, ensuring patient care is covered by a colleague.

Afternoon: Continued Care and Monitoring (1:00 PM - 4:00 PM)

- **Reassessments and Documentation:**

    - Reassess patients, particularly those who are unstable or have undergone procedures.

    - Monitor for any changes in condition and document ongoing care.

- **Handling Acute Changes:**
  - Respond to any urgent or emergent situations, such as a patient experiencing chest pain, a fall, or signs of sepsis.
  - Initiate appropriate interventions and escalate care if needed.

Late Afternoon: Pre-Shift Handoff Preparation (4:00 PM - 6:00 PM)

- **Winding Down:**
  - Begin preparing for the shift change by ensuring that all documentation is up to date.
  - Perform a final round of patient assessments and ensure that all care needs have been met.

- **Handoff Report:**
  - Prepare and give a detailed handoff to the incoming nurse, covering patient status, pending labs or procedures, and any significant events from the shift.

Shift End: (6:30 PM - 7:00 PM)

- **Final Tasks:**
  - Complete any last-minute tasks, such as ensuring patients are comfortable and that all equipment is properly stored and cleaned.
  - Clock out and attend a post-shift debrief if needed.

After Shift: Documentation and Self-Care

- **Final Documentation:**
  - If needed, finish any outstanding documentation before leaving the unit.

- **Self-Care:**
    - Transition out of work mode by relaxing, hydrating, and preparing for the next day's shift.

This is a general outline, and the specific details can vary depending on the unit's specialty (e.g., med-surg, ICU, ortho trauma) and patient load. Acute care nurses must be flexible and prepared to adjust their workflow based on patient needs and unexpected events.

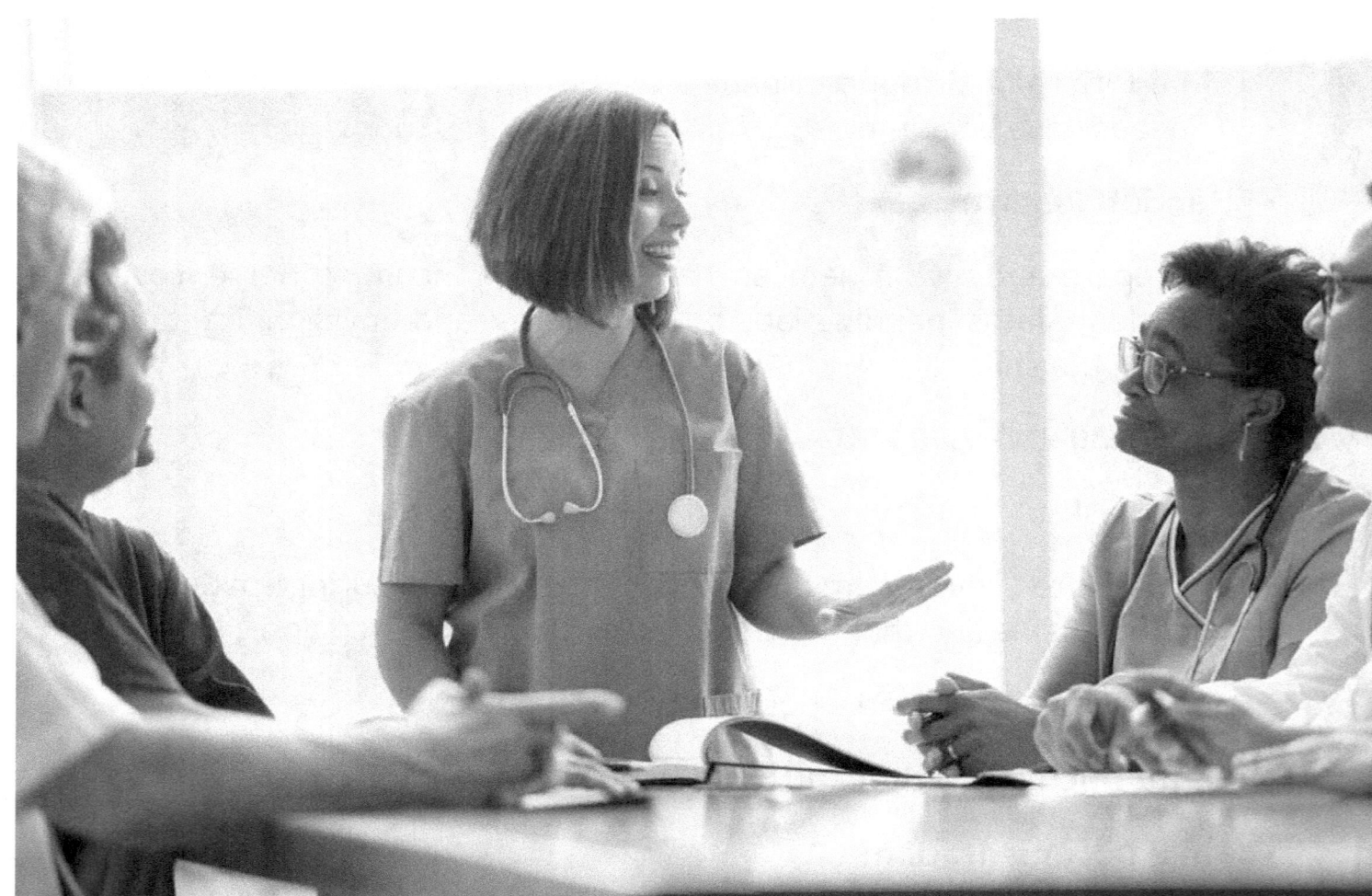

Assessment & Management of Patient Conditions By Body System

Circulatory System

Circulatory conditions affect the heart and blood vessels and can impact overall cardiovascular health. Here are some common circulatory conditions:

1. **Hypertension (High Blood Pressure):**

   - **Description:** A chronic condition where blood pressure in the arteries is consistently elevated.

   - **Symptoms:** Often asymptomatic; can cause headaches, dizziness, and shortness of breath.

   - **Complications:** Can lead to heart disease, stroke, kidney damage, and vision loss.

   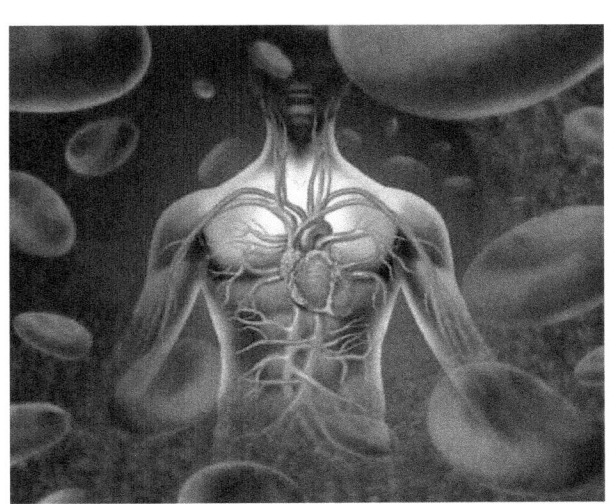

2. **Coronary Artery Disease (CAD):**

   - **Description:** A condition where the coronary arteries are narrowed or blocked due to plaque buildup.

   - **Symptoms:** Chest pain (angina), shortness of breath, fatigue.

   - **Complications:** Can lead to heart attacks (myocardial infarctions).

3. **Heart Failure:**

   - **Description:** A condition where the heart is unable to pump blood effectively to meet the body's needs.

   - **Symptoms:** Shortness of breath, fatigue, swollen legs and ankles, rapid or irregular heartbeat.

- **Complications:** Can lead to fluid buildup in the lungs or other parts of the body.

4. **Arrhythmias:**
    - **Description:** Abnormal heart rhythms that can affect the heart's ability to pump blood efficiently.
    - **Types:** Includes atrial fibrillation, ventricular tachycardia, and bradycardia.
    - **Symptoms:** Palpitations, dizziness, fainting, shortness of breath.

5. **Peripheral Artery Disease (PAD):**
    - **Description:** A condition where narrowed arteries reduce blood flow to the limbs.
    - **Symptoms:** Pain or cramping in the legs during physical activity (claudication), numbness, weakness.
    - **Complications:** Can lead to non-healing wounds or ulcers and increase the risk of heart attack or stroke.

6. **Deep Vein Thrombosis (DVT):**
    - **Description:** Formation of a blood clot in a deep vein, usually in the legs.
    - **Symptoms:** Swelling, pain, redness, or warmth in the affected leg.
    - **Complications:** Can lead to pulmonary embolism if the clot dislodges and travels to the lungs.

7. **Varicose Veins:**
    - **Description:** Enlarged, twisted veins usually found in the legs.
    - **Symptoms:** Aching pain, heaviness, and swelling in the legs.
    - **Complications:** Can lead to skin ulcers or blood clots.

8. **Aneurysms:**

    - **Description:** Abnormal bulges in the walls of blood vessels, most commonly the aorta.

    - **Symptoms:** Often asymptomatic; can cause pain or discomfort if large.

    - **Complications:** Can lead to rupture, causing severe bleeding and potentially life-threatening conditions.

9. **Myocarditis:**

    - **Description:** Inflammation of the heart muscle, often caused by a viral infection.

    - **Symptoms:** Chest pain, fatigue, shortness of breath, and swelling in the legs.

    - **Complications:** Can lead to heart failure or sudden cardiac death.

10. **Endocarditis:**

    - **Description:** Infection of the inner lining of the heart chambers and valves.

    - **Symptoms:** Fever, chills, fatigue, and heart murmur.

    - **Complications:** Can damage heart valves and lead to heart failure or embolic events.

These conditions require prompt diagnosis and management to prevent complications and maintain cardiovascular health.

Digestive System

Conditions

1. **Acute Gastroenteritis:**

   - **Assessment:** Monitor for symptoms such as diarrhea, vomiting, abdominal pain, and dehydration.
   - **Hydration:** Administer IV fluids and electrolytes to address dehydration.
   - **Medications:** Provide antiemetics or antidiarrheals as prescribed.
   - **Monitoring:** Regularly assess vital signs, fluid intake and output, and electrolyte levels.

2. **Appendicitis:**

   - **Assessment:** Monitor for symptoms such as right lower quadrant pain, nausea, vomiting, and fever.
   - **Surgical Intervention:** Prepare the patient for appendectomy and provide preoperative care.
   - **Pain Management:** Administer analgesics as prescribed.
   - **Monitoring:** Monitor for signs of complications, such as peritonitis or sepsis.

3. **Peptic Ulcer Disease:**

   - **Assessment:** Monitor for symptoms like epigastric pain, nausea, vomiting, and melena.
   - **Medications:** Administer proton pump inhibitors (PPIs), H2-receptor antagonists, or antibiotics if H. pylori infection is present.
   - **Supportive Care:** Provide pain management and educate on dietary modifications.
   - **Monitoring:** Assess for signs of gastrointestinal bleeding or perforation.

4. **Gastrointestinal Bleeding:**

    - **Assessment:** Monitor for symptoms such as hematemesis (vomiting blood), melena (black tarry stools), or hematochezia (bright red blood in stools).

    - **Interventions:** Administer IV fluids, blood products, and medications as prescribed. Prepare for endoscopy or surgery if needed.

    - **Monitoring:** Regularly assess vital signs, hemoglobin levels, and signs of hypovolemic shock.

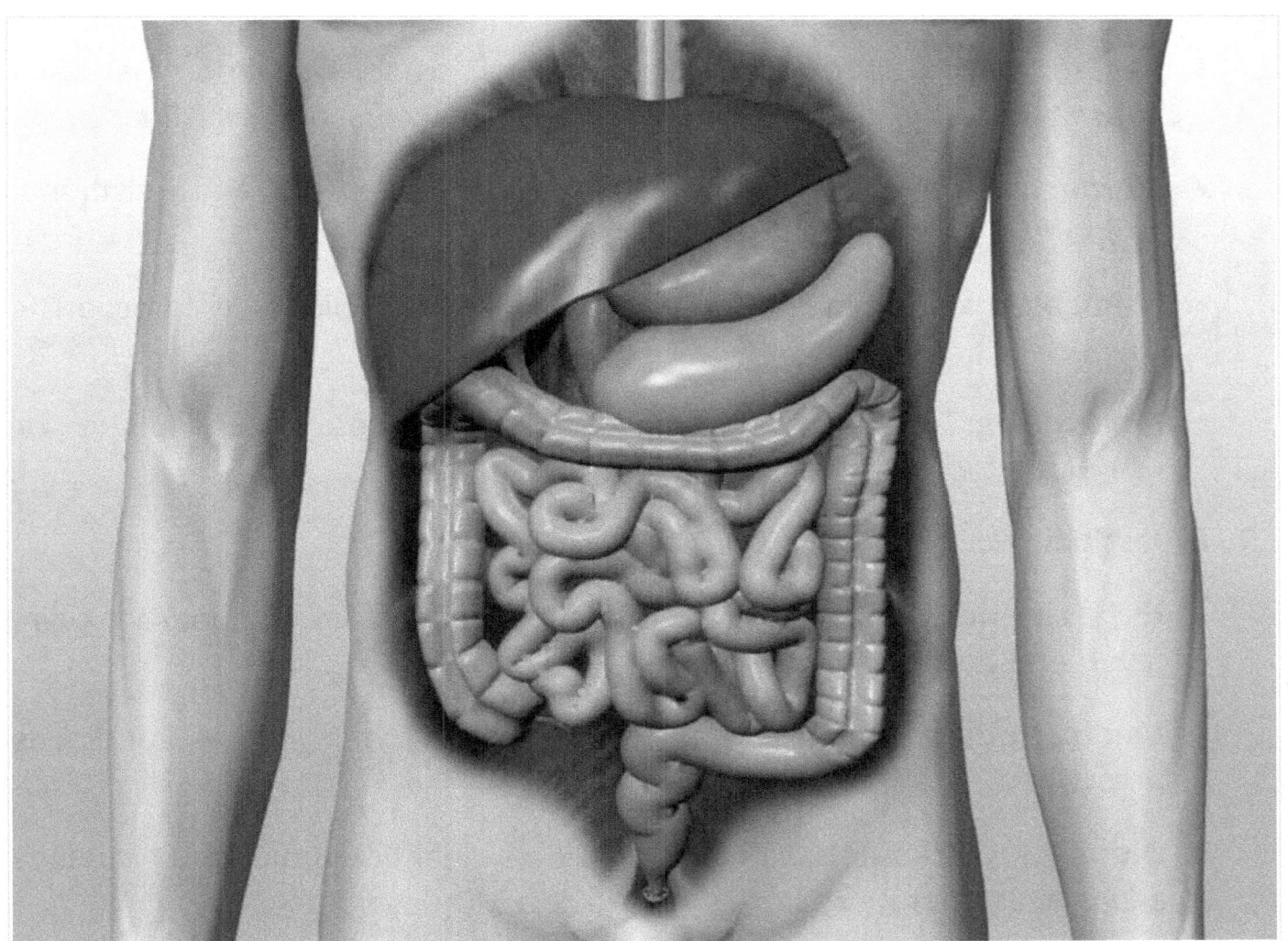

5. **Cholecystitis:**
   - **Assessment:** Monitor for symptoms such as right upper quadrant pain, fever, and nausea.
   - **Medications:** Administer analgesics and antibiotics as prescribed.
   - **Surgical Intervention:** Prepare for cholecystectomy if indicated.
   - **Monitoring:** Monitor for signs of complications such as gallbladder perforation or pancreatitis.

6. **Pancreatitis:**
   - **Assessment:** Monitor for symptoms such as severe abdominal pain, nausea, vomiting, and elevated pancreatic enzymes (amylase, lipase).
   - **Supportive Care:** Provide IV fluids, pain management, and nutritional support.
   - **Medications:** Administer pain relievers and antibiotics if infection is suspected.
   - **Monitoring:** Assess for complications such as organ failure or pseudocyst formation.

7. **Diverticulitis:**
   - **Assessment:** Monitor for symptoms such as left lower quadrant pain, fever, and changes in bowel habits.
   - **Medications:** Administer antibiotics and pain management as prescribed.
   - **Dietary Modifications:** Initially, provide a clear liquid diet and gradually advance as tolerated. Diet's still require a MD order.
   - **Monitoring:** Monitor for signs of complications such as perforation or abscess formation.

8. **Bowel Obstruction:**
   - **Assessment:** Monitor for symptoms such as abdominal pain, distension, vomiting, and changes in bowel movements.
   - **Interventions:** Administer IV fluids, correct electrolyte imbalances, and prepare for potential surgical intervention.
   - **Monitoring:** Regularly assess bowel sounds, abdominal girth, and response to treatment.

9. **Inflammatory Bowel Disease (IBD) (e.g., Crohn's Disease, Ulcerative Colitis):**
   - **Assessment:** Monitor for symptoms such as abdominal pain, diarrhea, weight loss, and signs of dehydration.
   - **Medications:** Administer anti-inflammatory medications, immunosuppressants, or biologics as prescribed.
   - **Supportive Care:** Provide nutritional support and manage symptoms.
   - **Monitoring:** Assess for complications such as bowel perforation or fistula formation.

10. **Hepatitis:**
    - **Assessment:** Monitor for symptoms such as jaundice, abdominal pain, and elevated liver enzymes.
    - **Supportive Care:** Provide nutritional support and manage symptoms.
    - **Medications:** Administer antiviral or other medications as prescribed.
    - **Monitoring:** Regularly assess liver function tests and monitor for signs of liver failure.

11. **Cirrhosis:**

    - **Assessment:** Monitor for symptoms such as ascites, jaundice, and confusion (hepatic encephalopathy).

    - **Interventions:** Provide diuretics for ascites, manage electrolyte imbalances, and administer lactulose for hepatic encephalopathy.

    - **Monitoring:** Regularly assess liver function, fluid status, and signs of complications such as variceal bleeding.

12. **Esophageal Varices:**

    - **Assessment:** Monitor for symptoms such as hematemesis, melena, and signs of portal hypertension.

    - **Interventions:** Provide supportive care, administer vasoconstrictors, and prepare for possible endoscopic intervention or balloon tamponade.

    - **Monitoring:** Regularly assess vital signs, signs of bleeding, and response to treatment.

13. **Hiatal Hernia:**

    - **Assessment:** Monitor for symptoms such as acid reflux, chest pain, and difficulty swallowing.

    - **Medications:** Administer proton pump inhibitors (PPIs) or H2-receptor antagonists to manage acid reflux.

    - **Dietary Modifications:** Provide guidance on dietary changes to reduce symptoms.

    - **Monitoring:** Assess response to medications and dietary changes.

These conditions require careful monitoring, timely interventions, and coordination with other healthcare professionals to manage acute digestive issues and support patient recovery.

Endocrine-These conditions often involve hormonal imbalances that affect various body systems

1. **Diabetic Ketoacidosis (DKA):**

   - **Assessment:** Monitor for symptoms such as hyperglycemia, ketonuria, acidosis (elevated anion gap), and signs of dehydration.

   - **Interventions:**
     - **Fluid Replacement:** Administer IV fluids to correct dehydration and electrolyte imbalances.
     - **Insulin Therapy:** Administer insulin to lower blood glucose levels.
     - **Electrolyte Monitoring:** Monitor and replace electrolytes, particularly potassium.

   - **Monitoring:** Regularly check blood glucose, ketone levels, and arterial blood gases (ABGs).

2. **Hyperosmolar Hyperglycemic State (HHS):**

   - **Assessment:** Monitor for symptoms such as extreme hyperglycemia, dehydration, altered mental status, and electrolyte imbalances.

   - **Interventions:**
     - **Fluid Replacement:** Administer IV fluids to correct dehydration.
     - **Insulin Therapy:** Administer insulin to reduce blood glucose levels.
     - **Electrolyte Monitoring:** Regularly monitor and replace electrolytes.

   - **Monitoring:** Continuously assess blood glucose levels, fluid status, and mental status.

3. **Thyroid Storm:**

    - **Assessment:** Monitor for symptoms such as fever, tachycardia, agitation, and confusion.

    - **Interventions:**

        - **Antithyroid Medications:** Administer medications to inhibit thyroid hormone production (e.g., methimazole, propylthiouracil).

        - **Supportive Care:** Provide supportive care including cooling measures, and beta-blockers to manage symptoms.

        - **Hydration and Electrolytes:** Administer IV fluids and monitor electrolytes.

    - **Monitoring:** Regularly assess vital signs, thyroid function tests, and response to treatment.

4. **Myxedema Coma:**

    - **Assessment:** Monitor for symptoms such as severe hypothyroidism, hypothermia, altered mental status, and bradycardia.

    - **Interventions:**

        - **Thyroid Hormone Replacement:** Administer IV levothyroxine.

        - **Supportive Care:** Provide warming measures and supportive care.

        - **Hydration and Electrolytes:** Administer IV fluids and monitor electrolytes.

    - **Monitoring:** Regularly check thyroid function tests and vital signs.

5. Adrenal Crisis:

- **Assessment:** Monitor for symptoms such as severe fatigue, hypotension, hypoglycemia, and electrolyte imbalances.
- **Interventions:**
    - **Glucocorticoid Replacement:** Administer IV hydrocortisone or other glucocorticoids.
    - **Fluid Replacement:** Administer IV fluids to manage hypotension and dehydration.
    - **Electrolyte Monitoring:** Monitor and correct electrolyte imbalances, especially sodium and potassium.
- **Monitoring:** Continuously monitor vital signs, electrolyte levels, and response to treatment.

6. Pheochromocytoma Crisis:

- **Assessment:** Monitor for symptoms such as severe hypertension, tachycardia, headache, and sweating.
- **Interventions:**
    - **Alpha-Blockade:** Administer alpha-adrenergic blockers to manage hypertension.
    - **Fluid Replacement:** Provide IV fluids if needed to manage blood pressure.
    - **Prepare for Surgery:** Coordinate with surgical teams for potential tumor removal.
- **Monitoring:** Regularly check blood pressure, heart rate, and response to medications.

7. **Hyperparathyroidism Crisis:**

   - **Assessment:** Monitor for symptoms such as hypercalcemia, confusion, abdominal pain, and kidney stones.

   - **Interventions:**

     - **Hydration:** Administer IV fluids to help lower calcium levels and prevent kidney damage.

     - **Medications:** Administer medications such as bisphosphonates or calcitonin to lower calcium levels.

   - **Monitoring:** Regularly assess calcium levels, renal function, and vital signs.

8. **Hypoparathyroidism Crisis:**

   - **Assessment:** Monitor for symptoms such as hypocalcemia, tetany, seizures, and muscle cramps.

   - **Interventions:**

     - **Calcium Replacement:** Administer IV calcium gluconate or calcium chloride.

     - **Vitamin D Supplementation:** Provide vitamin D supplements to aid calcium absorption.

     - **Monitor:** Regularly check calcium and phosphate levels, as well as signs of hypocalcemia.

   - **Monitoring:** Continuously assess vital signs and response to treatment.

9. **Diabetic Foot Ulcers:**

- **Assessment:** Monitor for signs of infection, tissue damage, and non-healing ulcers in patients with diabetes.

- **Interventions:**

    - **Wound Care:** Provide proper wound care, including debridement and dressing changes.

    - **Infection Control:** Administer antibiotics as needed and manage glycemic control.

    - **Pressure Relief:** Provide measures to relieve pressure on the affected foot.

- **Monitoring:** Regularly assess wound healing, infection signs, and glycemic control.

10. **Cushing's Syndrome:**

- **Assessment:** Monitor for symptoms such as hypertension, weight gain, and hyperglycemia.

- **Interventions:**

    - **Medications:** Administer medications to control cortisol production if indicated.

    - **Supportive Care:** Manage symptoms and provide supportive care.

- **Monitoring:** Regularly assess cortisol levels, blood pressure, and glucose levels.

11. **Addison's Disease:**

    - **Assessment:** Monitor for symptoms such as fatigue, weight loss, and hyperpigmentation.

    - **Interventions:**

        - **Hormone Replacement:** Administer glucocorticoids and mineralocorticoids as needed.

        - **Hydration:** Provide IV fluids if needed to manage blood pressure and dehydration.

    - **Monitoring:** Regularly assess adrenal hormone levels, electrolyte balance, and vital signs.

These conditions require timely assessment and management to stabilize the patient and address acute symptoms, prevent complications, and support recovery.

Immune System

1. **Sepsis:**

    - **Assessment:** Monitor for signs of systemic infection, such as fever, chills, rapid heart rate, hypotension, and altered mental status.

    - **Interventions:**

        - **Antibiotics:** Administer broad-spectrum antibiotics as soon as possible.

        - **Fluid Resuscitation:** Provide IV fluids to address hypotension and maintain blood pressure.

        - **Vasopressors:** Administer medications to stabilize blood pressure if needed.

    - **Monitoring:** Continuously monitor vital signs, lactate levels, and organ function.

2. **Systemic Lupus Erythematosus (SLE) Flare:**

   - **Assessment:** Monitor for symptoms such as joint pain, rash, fever, and signs of organ involvement (e.g., renal impairment).
   - **Interventions:**
     - **Medications:** Administer corticosteroids or immunosuppressants as prescribed.
     - **Supportive Care:** Provide pain management and address any complications (e.g., renal issues).
   - **Monitoring:** Regularly assess vital signs, renal function, and response to medications.

3. **Rheumatoid Arthritis Flare:**

   - **Assessment:** Monitor for joint pain, swelling, and stiffness, as well as systemic symptoms such as fever.
   - **Interventions:**
     - **Medications:** Administer corticosteroids, disease-modifying antirheumatic drugs (DMARDs), or biologics as prescribed.
     - **Supportive Care:** Provide pain management and physical therapy if needed.
   - **Monitoring:** Regularly assess joint function and response to treatment.

4. **Anaphylaxis:**

   - **Assessment:** Monitor for signs of severe allergic reaction, such as difficulty breathing, swelling of the face or throat, hives, and hypotension.
   - **Interventions:**
     - **Epinephrine:** Administer intramuscular epinephrine immediately.
     - **Oxygen Therapy:** Provide supplemental oxygen if needed.

- **Antihistamines and Steroids:** Administer antihistamines and corticosteroids to reduce inflammation and allergic response.
- **Monitoring:** Continuously monitor vital signs and patient response to treatment.

5. **Autoimmune Hemolytic Anemia:**
    - **Assessment:** Monitor for symptoms such as fatigue, pallor, jaundice, and signs of hemolysis.
    - **Interventions:**
        - **Blood Transfusion:** Administer packed red blood cells if anemia is severe.
        - **Medications:** Provide corticosteroids or immunosuppressants as prescribed.
    - **Monitoring:** Regularly assess hemoglobin levels, reticulocyte count, and response to treatment.

6. **Immunocompromised States (e.g., HIV/AIDS):**
    - **Assessment:** Monitor for opportunistic infections, weight loss, and symptoms related to specific infections (e.g., pneumocystis pneumonia).
    - **Interventions:**
        - **Antiretroviral Therapy:** Administer ART to manage HIV infection.
        - **Prophylactic Medications:** Provide prophylaxis for opportunistic infections as needed.
    - **Monitoring:** Regularly assess viral load, CD4 count, and response to treatment.

7. **Graft-Versus-Host Disease (GVHD):**

   - **Assessment:** Monitor for symptoms such as rash, diarrhea, and liver dysfunction following a bone marrow transplant.

   - **Interventions:**

     - **Immunosuppressants:** Administer medications to suppress the immune response, such as corticosteroids or calcineurin inhibitors.

     - **Supportive Care:** Provide supportive care to manage symptoms and prevent complications.

   - **Monitoring:** Regularly assess skin, gastrointestinal, and liver function.

8. **Primary Immunodeficiency Disorders:**

   - **Assessment:** Monitor for recurrent infections or unusual infections due to an underlying immune deficiency.

   - **Interventions:**

     - **Immunoglobulin Replacement:** Administer intravenous immunoglobulin (IVIG) if indicated.

     - **Antibiotics:** Provide prophylactic or therapeutic antibiotics as needed.

   - **Monitoring:** Regularly assess immune function and response to treatment.

9. **Vasculitis:**

   - **Assessment:** Monitor for symptoms such as systemic symptoms (fever, malaise), rash, and organ involvement (e.g., kidney or lung damage).

   - **Interventions:**

     - **Medications:** Administer corticosteroids or immunosuppressants as prescribed.

     - **Supportive Care:** Provide supportive care for symptoms and complications.

   - **Monitoring:** Regularly assess organ function, inflammatory markers, and response to treatment.

10. **Hyperacute Rejection of Transplants:**

    - **Assessment:** Monitor for immediate rejection symptoms such as fever, pain at the transplant site, and loss of organ function.

    - **Interventions:**

      - **Immunosuppressants:** Administer high-dose corticosteroids or other immunosuppressive agents.

      - **Supportive Care:** Provide supportive care and address any complications.

    - **Monitoring:** Regularly assess organ function and response to treatment.

These conditions require careful monitoring and prompt intervention to manage symptoms, prevent complications, and support overall patient health.

Integumentary System

Conditions

1. **Pressure Ulcers (Bedsores):**

    - **Assessment:** Regularly assess skin for redness, breakdown, or ulcers, especially in high-risk areas like heels, sacrum, and buttocks.

    - **Wound Care:** Clean and dress wounds as per protocol. Use appropriate wound care products and techniques.

    - **Pressure Relief:** Reposition the patient regularly to alleviate pressure on at-risk areas. Use specialized mattresses or cushions.

    - **Nutritional Support:** Ensure adequate nutrition and hydration to promote wound healing.

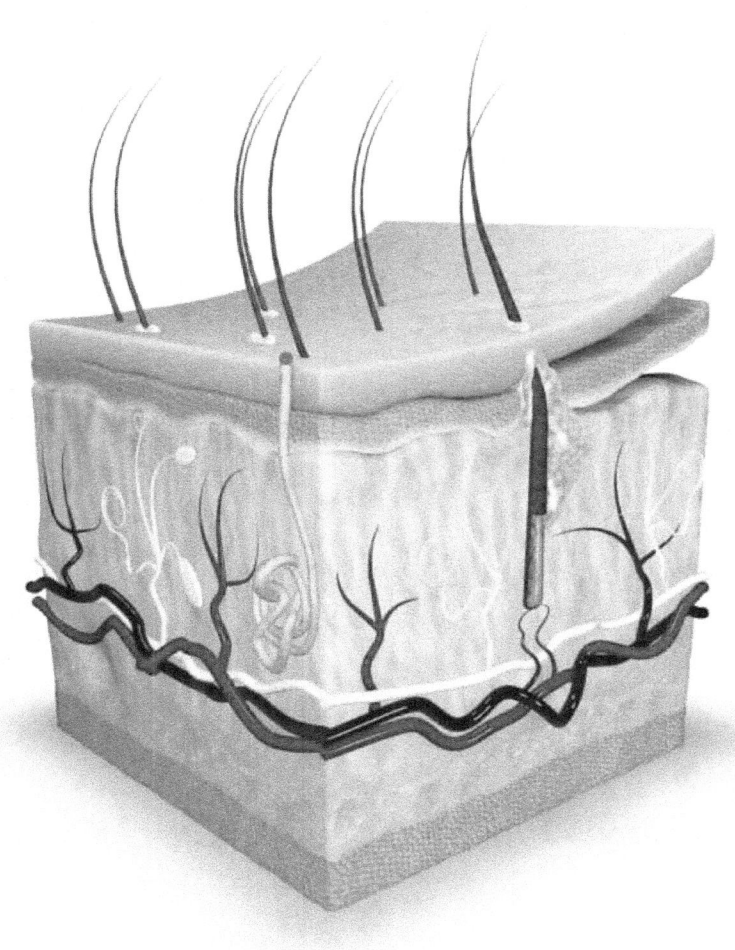

2. **Burns:**
   - **Assessment:** Evaluate the depth and extent of the burns (e.g., superficial, partial-thickness, full-thickness).
   - **Fluid Resuscitation:** Administer IV fluids to prevent shock and maintain hydration, following the Parkland formula or other protocols.
   - **Wound Care:** Cleanse and dress burns with appropriate materials (e.g., silver sulfadiazine) to prevent infection.
   - **Pain Management:** Provide analgesics and monitor pain levels frequently.
   - **Infection Prevention:** Monitor for signs of infection and implement strict infection control measures.

3. **Cellulitis:**
   - **Assessment:** Monitor for signs of redness, warmth, swelling, and pain in the affected area.
   - **Antibiotic Therapy:** Administer prescribed antibiotics to treat bacterial infections.
   - **Elevation:** Elevate the affected limb to reduce swelling and improve circulation.
   - **Pain Management:** Provide analgesics to manage pain and discomfort.

4. **Abscesses:**
   - **Assessment:** Assess for signs of localized swelling, redness, and tenderness.
   - **Drainage:** Assist with or perform incision and drainage (I&D) procedures as ordered.
   - **Antibiotic Therapy:** Administer antibiotics as prescribed to address the underlying infection.

- **Wound Care:** Provide proper wound care post-drainage to facilitate healing.

5. **Skin Infections (e.g., Impetigo, Herpes Simplex):**

    - **Assessment:** Monitor for lesions, blisters, or crusted sores.

    - **Antiviral or Antibacterial Treatment:** Administer medications as prescribed.

    - **Hygiene:** Implement strict hand hygiene and isolation precautions to prevent spread.

    - **Wound Care:** Clean and dress lesions as needed to promote healing.

6. **Eczema (Atopic Dermatitis):**

    - **Assessment:** Observe for redness, itching, and skin thickening or cracking.

    - **Topical Treatments:** Apply prescribed topical corticosteroids or emollients to manage inflammation and itching.

    - **Avoid Triggers:** Educate patients on avoiding known irritants and maintaining skin hydration.

7. **Psoriasis:**

    - **Assessment:** Monitor for plaques, scaling, and redness, typically found on the scalp, elbows, and knees.

    - **Topical Treatments:** Apply topical treatments such as corticosteroids or vitamin D analogs.

    - **Systemic Therapy:** Administer systemic medications (e.g., methotrexate, biologics) if prescribed.

    - **Moisturization:** Encourage regular use of moisturizers to reduce dryness and scaling.

8. **Skin Cancer (e.g., Melanoma, Basal Cell Carcinoma):**

    - **Assessment:** Assess for new or changing skin lesions, including changes in size, shape, or color.
    - **Biopsy:** Assist with or prepare for biopsy procedures to confirm diagnosis.
    - **Wound Care:** Provide care for surgical sites post-excision.

9. **Alopecia:**

    - **Assessment:** Monitor for hair loss patterns and any associated symptoms.
    - **Supportive Care:** Provide emotional support and education about potential treatment options.
    - **Treatment:** Assist with or administer prescribed treatments (e.g., corticosteroids for autoimmune alopecia).

10. **Dermatitis:**

    - **Assessment:** Look for signs of inflammation, itching, redness, or rash.
    - **Topical Treatment:** Apply prescribed topical medications or emollients.
    - **Avoid Irritants:** Educate patients on avoiding known irritants and using gentle skin care products.

These conditions require careful monitoring, timely interventions, and patient education to manage effectively and promote healing.

Muscular System

1. **Muscle Strains and Sprains:**

    - **Assessment:** Assess for pain, swelling, bruising, and limited range of motion in the affected area.

    - **Rest and Immobilization:** Provide support and immobilization to prevent further injury.

    - **Ice and Compression:** Apply ice and compression to reduce swelling and pain.

    - **Pain Management:** Administer analgesics and anti-inflammatory medications as prescribed.

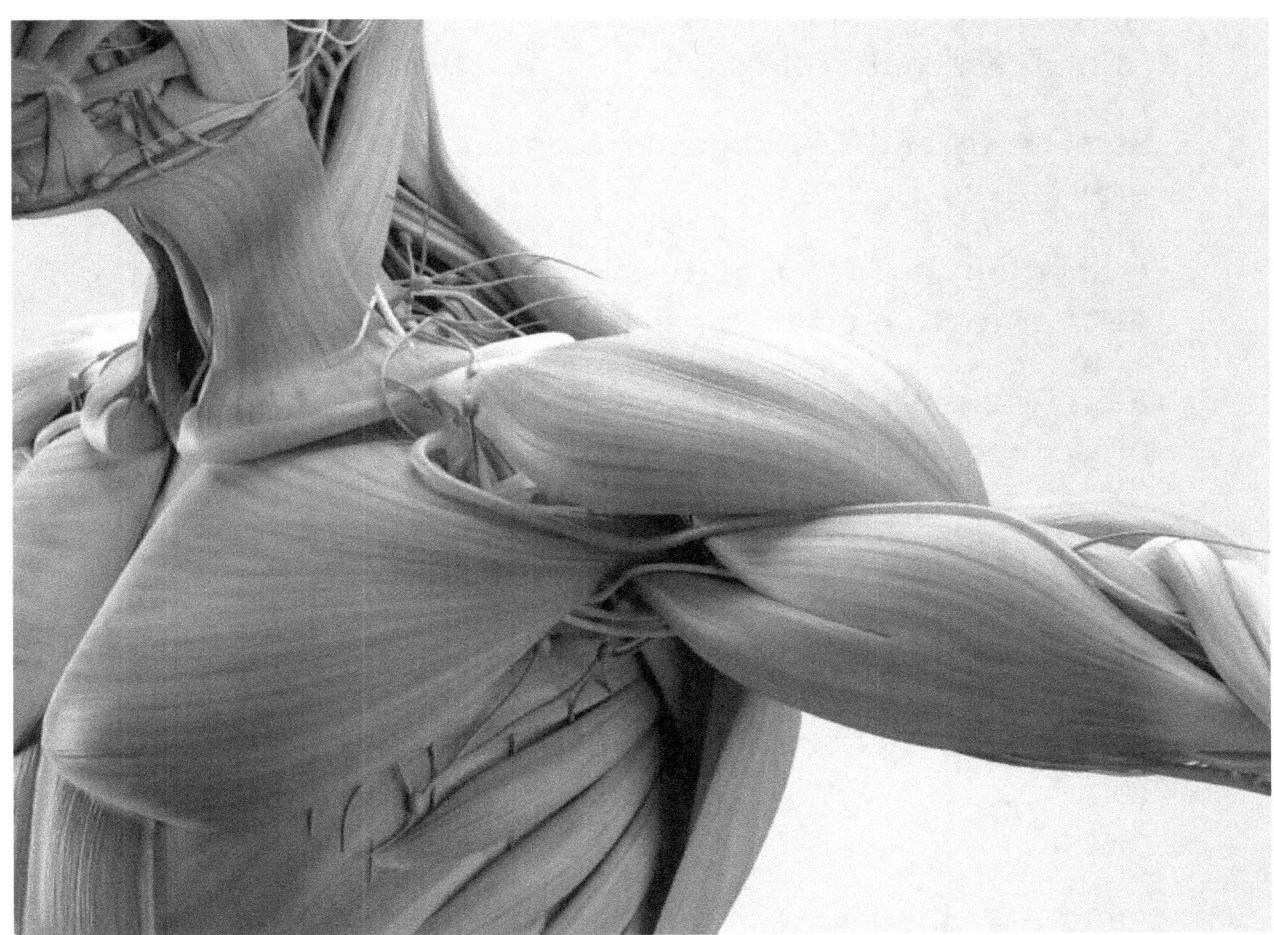

2. **Rhabdomyolysis:**
   - **Assessment:** Monitor for symptoms such as muscle pain, weakness, swelling, and dark urine.
   - **Hydration:** Administer IV fluids to maintain hydration and flush out toxins.
   - **Electrolyte Monitoring:** Regularly monitor and correct electrolyte imbalances, especially potassium levels.
   - **Renal Function:** Monitor kidney function closely for signs of acute kidney injury.

3. **Muscle Spasms and Cramps:**
   - **Assessment:** Evaluate for sudden onset of muscle pain, tightness, or involuntary contractions.
   - **Stretching and Massage:** Provide gentle stretching and massage to alleviate muscle spasms.
   - **Hydration and Electrolytes:** Ensure adequate hydration and monitor electrolytes to prevent imbalances.
   - **Pain Management:** Administer analgesics or muscle relaxants as prescribed.

4. **Compartment Syndrome:**
   - **Assessment:** Monitor for symptoms such as severe pain, swelling, and decreased sensation or movement in the affected limb.
   - **Immediate Action:** Elevate the limb and avoid applying ice or compression. Notify the healthcare provider urgently for possible fasciotomy.
   - **Pain Management:** Administer analgesics and monitor for effectiveness.

5. **Myopathy:**
   - **Assessment:** Assess for muscle weakness, pain, or stiffness, and evaluate muscle strength and function.
   - **Medication Management:** Administer prescribed medications, such as corticosteroids or immunosuppressants, as ordered.
   - **Physical Therapy:** Provide or coordinate physical therapy to maintain muscle function and mobility.

6. **Muscular Dystrophy:**
   - **Assessment:** Monitor for muscle weakness, wasting, and impaired mobility.
   - **Supportive Care:** Provide supportive care to manage symptoms and improve quality of life.
   - **Assistive Devices:** Assist with or provide adaptive devices to enhance mobility and independence.

7. **Tendon Injuries:**
   - **Assessment:** Evaluate for pain, swelling, and inability to move the affected joint or muscle.
   - **Immobilization:** Provide support and immobilization of the affected tendon.
   - **Surgical Intervention:** Prepare the patient for possible surgical repair if indicated.

8. **Spinal Cord Injuries:**
   - **Assessment:** Assess for muscle weakness, paralysis, or loss of sensation below the level of injury.
   - **Stabilization:** Ensure proper spinal immobilization and stabilization.
   - **Neurogenic Shock:** Monitor for signs of neurogenic shock and manage accordingly.

- **Rehabilitation:** Coordinate with physical therapy and rehabilitation services for ongoing care.

9. **Myositis:**

    - **Assessment:** Monitor for muscle inflammation, pain, and weakness.
    - **Medication:** Administer anti-inflammatory or immunosuppressive medications as prescribed.
    - **Physical Therapy:** Provide or coordinate physical therapy to maintain muscle strength and function.

10. **Fibromyalgia:**

    - **Assessment:** Evaluate for widespread musculoskeletal pain, fatigue, and tender points.
    - **Pain Management:** Administer analgesics, antidepressants, or muscle relaxants as prescribed.
    - **Patient Education:** Educate the patient on managing symptoms and incorporating stress-reducing activities.

11. **Tetanus:**

    - **Assessment:** Monitor for symptoms such as muscle stiffness, spasms, and difficulty swallowing.
    - **Tetanus Immunization:** Administer tetanus immunoglobulin and/or booster vaccine as indicated.
    - **Supportive Care:** Provide supportive care to manage muscle spasms and prevent complications.

These interventions aim to manage pain, prevent complications, and support recovery for patients with muscular system conditions in an acute care setting.

Nervous System

1. **Stroke (Cerebrovascular Accident):**

    - **Assessment:** Evaluate for sudden onset of symptoms such as facial droop, arm weakness, speech difficulties, or confusion.

    - **Imaging:** Facilitate rapid imaging (CT/MRI) to determine the type and extent of the stroke.

    - **Medication Administration:** Administer thrombolytics or anticoagulants as prescribed, depending on the type of stroke.

    - **Monitoring:** Continuously monitor neurological status, vital signs, and for signs of complications such as bleeding.

    - **Supportive Care:** Assist with swallowing and mobility issues, and coordinate rehabilitation services.

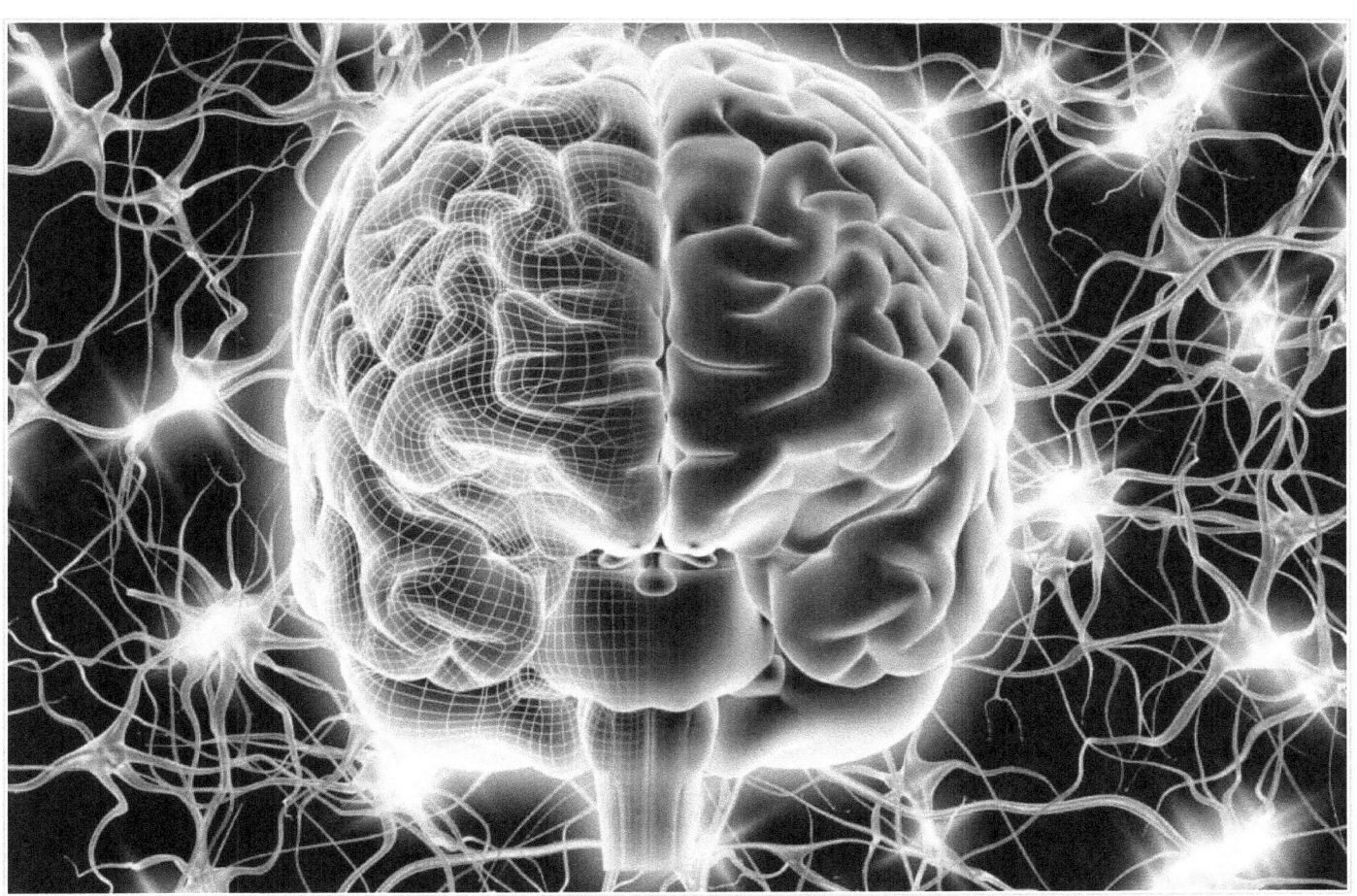

2. **Seizures:**
   - **Assessment:** Observe and document seizure activity, including duration, type, and any postictal symptoms.
   - **Seizure Precautions:** Implement safety measures to prevent injury, such as padding bed rails.
   - **Medication Administration:** Administer anticonvulsants as prescribed and monitor for effectiveness and side effects.
   - **Monitoring:** Monitor vital signs, neurological status, and for potential causes or triggers of seizures.

3. **Head Injury/Traumatic Brain Injury (TBI):**
   - **Assessment:** Monitor for changes in consciousness, pupil reactions, and neurological deficits.
   - **Imaging:** Ensure timely imaging (CT/MRI) to assess for intracranial bleeding or swelling.
   - **Monitoring:** Regularly monitor intracranial pressure (ICP) if applicable, and vital signs.
   - **Supportive Care:** Provide appropriate positioning and minimize stimulation to reduce ICP.

4. **Meningitis:**
   - **Assessment:** Observe for symptoms such as severe headache, neck stiffness, photophobia, and altered mental status.
   - **Medication Administration:** Administer antibiotics and antiviral medications as prescribed, and monitor for effectiveness.
   - **Isolation Precautions:** Implement droplet precautions if bacterial meningitis is suspected.
   - **Supportive Care:** Provide fever management, pain relief, and monitor for complications.

5. **Encephalitis:**

    - **Assessment:** Monitor for symptoms such as fever, headache, altered mental status, and seizures.

    - **Medication Administration:** Administer antiviral or antibiotic medications as prescribed based on the underlying cause.

    - **Supportive Care:** Provide supportive care including hydration, fever management, and monitoring for complications.

6. **Guillain-Barré Syndrome:**

    - **Assessment:** Monitor for progressive muscle weakness, paralysis, and respiratory function.

    - **Plasmapheresis or IVIG:** Administer plasmapheresis or intravenous immunoglobulin (IVIG) as ordered.

    - **Respiratory Support:** Prepare for and provide ventilatory support if needed.

    - **Physical Therapy:** Assist with or coordinate physical therapy to maintain muscle function and mobility.

7. **Myasthenia Gravis:**

    - **Assessment:** Monitor for muscle weakness, ptosis (drooping eyelids), and difficulty swallowing.

    - **Medication Administration:** Administer acetyl cholinesterase inhibitors or immune suppressants as prescribed.

    - **Crisis Management:** Prepare for potential myasthenic crisis or cholinergic crisis and provide appropriate interventions.

8. **Multiple Sclerosis (MS):**
   - **Assessment:** Monitor for exacerbations, including changes in vision, muscle strength, and coordination.
   - **Medication Administration:** Administer corticosteroids or disease-modifying therapies as prescribed.
   - **Supportive Care:** Provide supportive care to manage symptoms and coordinate rehabilitation services.

9. **Parkinson's Disease:**
   - **Assessment:** Monitor for symptoms such as tremors, rigidity, bradykinesia, and postural instability.
   - **Medication Administration:** Administer dopaminergic medications or other prescribed therapies.
   - **Physical Therapy:** Coordinate physical therapy to improve mobility and balance.

10. **Dementia:**
    - **Assessment:** Monitor for changes in cognition, memory, and behavior.
    - **Safety Measures:** Implement safety measures to prevent wandering or injury.
    - **Supportive Care:** Provide supportive care and coordinate with caregivers or social services for additional support.

11. **Neuropathy (e.g., Diabetic Neuropathy):**
    - **Assessment:** Assess for symptoms such as pain, numbness, or tingling in extremities.
    - **Pain Management:** Administer pain relief and manage symptoms as prescribed.
    - **Foot Care:** Provide education on proper foot care and monitoring for ulcers or injuries.

12. **Hydrocephalus:**

    - **Assessment:** Monitor for symptoms of increased intracranial pressure, such as headache, nausea, or changes in consciousness.

    - **Shunt Management:** Monitor and manage ventriculoperitoneal shunt function if applicable.

    - **Supportive Care:** Provide care to address symptoms and coordinate follow-up with neurosurgery if needed.

These interventions are aimed at stabilizing patients, preventing complications, and supporting recovery for those with nervous system conditions in an acute care setting.

Reproductive System

Conditions

1. Pregnancy-Related Complications:

- **Preterm Labor:**

    - **Assessment:** Monitor for signs of premature contractions, cervical changes, and fetal distress.

    - **Medications:** Administer tocolytics to delay preterm labor and corticosteroids for fetal lung maturation.

    - **Monitoring:** Track maternal and fetal vital signs and contractions.

- **Eclampsia/Preeclampsia:**

    - **Assessment:** Monitor for symptoms like hypertension, proteinuria, and seizures.

    - **Medications:** Administer antihypertensives and magnesium sulfate to prevent seizures.

    - **Monitoring:** Regularly check blood pressure, urine output, and fetal heart rate.

- **Gestational Diabetes:**
  - **Assessment:** Monitor blood glucose levels and assess for complications.
  - **Management:** Administer insulin or other glucose-lowering medications and provide dietary guidance.
  - **Monitoring:** Regularly check maternal and fetal blood glucose levels.

- **Placental Abruption/Placenta Previa:**
  - **Assessment:** Monitor for abnormal bleeding, abdominal pain, and fetal distress.
  - **Interventions:** Prepare for possible cesarean delivery and provide supportive care.
  - **Monitoring:** Regularly assess maternal vital signs, bleeding, and fetal heart rate.

2. Gynecological Emergencies:

- **Ovarian Cysts/Tumors:**
  - **Assessment:** Monitor for abdominal pain, bloating, or changes in menstrual cycles.
  - **Imaging:** Facilitate ultrasound or other imaging studies to assess cysts or tumors.
  - **Interventions:** Provide pain management and prepare for possible surgical intervention if indicated.

- **Pelvic Inflammatory Disease (PID):**
    - **Assessment:** Monitor for symptoms such as pelvic pain, fever, and abnormal discharge.
    - **Medications:** Administer broad-spectrum antibiotics to treat infection.
    - **Supportive Care:** Provide pain management and monitor for complications.
- **Ectopic Pregnancy:**
    - **Assessment:** Monitor for symptoms like abdominal pain, vaginal bleeding, and signs of shock.
    - **Treatment:** Administer medications (e.g., methotrexate) or prepare for surgical intervention if necessary.
    - **Monitoring:** Regularly assess vital signs and follow up with imaging studies.

3. Obstetric Emergencies:

- **Miscarriage (Spontaneous Abortion):**
    - **Assessment:** Monitor for bleeding, cramping, and passage of tissue.
    - **Supportive Care:** Provide emotional support, pain management, and prepare for possible surgical intervention if needed.
- **Postpartum Hemorrhage:**
    - **Assessment:** Monitor for excessive bleeding, changes in vital signs, and signs of shock.
    - **Interventions:** Administer uterotonics to promote uterine contraction and manage bleeding.
    - **Monitoring:** Regularly assess maternal vital signs, blood loss, and uterine tone.

- **Uterine Rupture:**
    - **Assessment:** Monitor for sudden onset of abdominal pain, fetal distress, and abnormal contractions.
    - **Interventions:** Prepare for emergency cesarean delivery and provide supportive care.
    - **Monitoring:** Continuously assess maternal and fetal vital signs and labor progress.

4. Sexually Transmitted Infections (STIs):

- **Assessment:** Monitor for symptoms such as discharge, pain, or sores.
- **Testing:** Perform diagnostic tests to identify the STI.
- **Medications:** Administer appropriate antibiotics or antivirals based on the STI.
- **Education:** Provide education on STI prevention and management.

5. Menstrual Disorders:

- **Heavy Menstrual Bleeding (Menorrhagia):**
    - **Assessment:** Monitor for excessive bleeding, anemia, and associated symptoms.
    - **Management:** Administer medications (e.g., hormonal therapies) or prepare for possible surgical interventions (e.g., dilation and curettage).
- **Amenorrhea:**
    - **Assessment:** Evaluate for underlying causes such as hormonal imbalances or stress.
    - **Management:** Provide treatment based on the underlying cause, including hormonal therapy or lifestyle modifications.

6. Prolapsed Organs:

- **Assessment:** Monitor for symptoms such as pelvic pressure, urinary incontinence, or difficulty with bowel movements.

- **Interventions:** Provide supportive care and prepare for possible surgical intervention if necessary.

These conditions often require prompt assessment and intervention to manage acute symptoms, prevent complications, and provide appropriate care and support for patients.

Respiratory System

Conditions

1. Chronic Obstructive Pulmonary Disease (COPD) Exacerbation:

- **Assessment:** Monitor for increased dyspnea, wheezing, productive cough, and changes in sputum color.

- **Oxygen Therapy:** Administer supplemental oxygen to maintain adequate oxygen saturation.

- **Medications:** Provide bronchodilators and corticosteroids as prescribed.

- **Monitoring:** Continuously monitor vital signs, respiratory status, and oxygen saturation.

2. Asthma Exacerbation:

- **Assessment:** Evaluate for symptoms such as wheezing, shortness of breath, chest tightness, and coughing.

- **Medications:** Administer bronchodilators (e.g., albuterol) and corticosteroids as ordered.

- **Oxygen Therapy:** Provide supplemental oxygen if needed to maintain adequate oxygen levels.

- **Monitoring:** Regularly monitor respiratory status and response to medications.

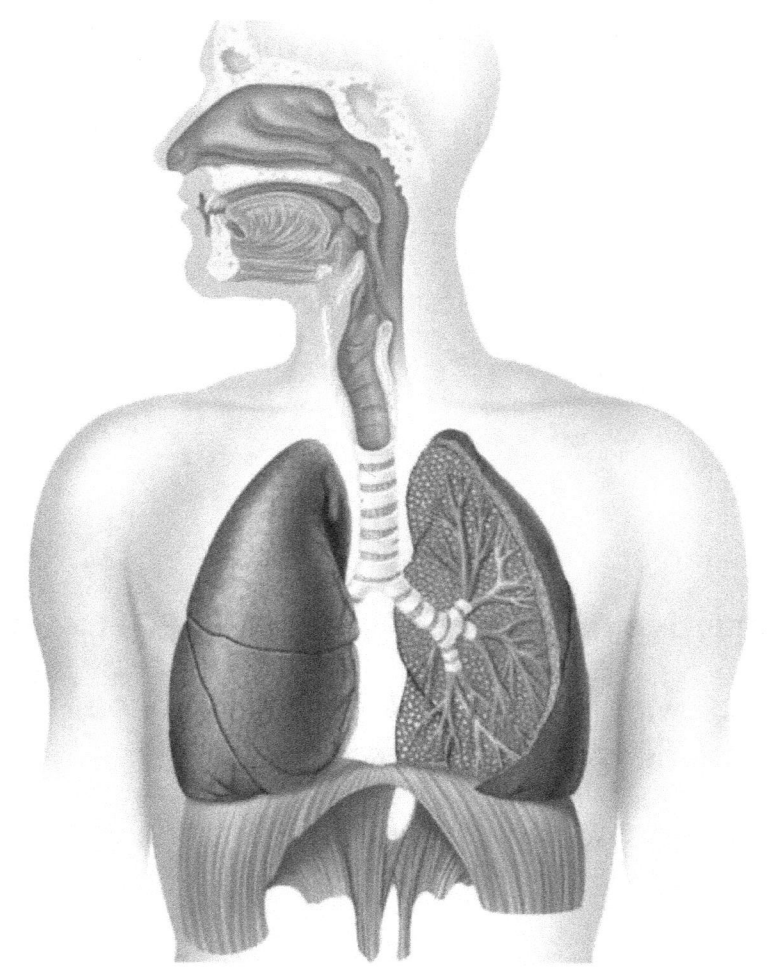

3. Pneumonia:

- **Assessment:** Monitor for symptoms such as fever, cough, sputum production, and chest pain.

- **Medications:** Administer antibiotics or antivirals based on the causative agent and local guidelines.

- **Oxygen Therapy:** Provide supplemental oxygen if needed.

- **Monitoring:** Assess respiratory status, vital signs, and response to treatment.

4. Pulmonary Embolism:

- **Assessment:** Monitor for symptoms such as sudden onset of shortness of breath, chest pain, and hypoxemia.
- **Medications:** Administer anticoagulants or thrombolytics as prescribed.
- **Oxygen Therapy:** Provide supplemental oxygen to maintain adequate oxygen saturation.
- **Monitoring:** Regularly assess vital signs, respiratory status, and response to treatment.

5. Acute Respiratory Distress Syndrome (ARDS):

- **Assessment:** Monitor for severe dyspnea, hypoxemia, and bilateral infiltrates on chest imaging.
- **Ventilator Support:** Provide mechanical ventilation with appropriate settings to support oxygenation and ventilation.
- **Prone Positioning:** Consider prone positioning to improve oxygenation.
- **Monitoring:** Continuously monitor respiratory status, oxygen saturation, and ventilation parameters.

6. Pleural Effusion:

- **Assessment:** Monitor for symptoms such as dyspnea, pleuritic chest pain, and decreased breath sounds.
- **Interventions:** Prepare for and assist with thoracentesis to remove excess fluid.
- **Oxygen Therapy:** Provide supplemental oxygen if necessary.
- **Monitoring:** Assess respiratory status and response to fluid removal.

7. **Pneumothorax:**

    - **Assessment:** Monitor for sudden onset of sharp chest pain, dyspnea, and decreased breath sounds on affected side.

    - **Interventions:** Prepare for and assist with chest tube insertion to evacuate air from the pleural space.

    - **Oxygen Therapy:** Provide supplemental oxygen to maintain adequate oxygen saturation.

    - **Monitoring:** Regularly assess respiratory status and chest tube function.

8. **Respiratory Failure:**

    - **Assessment:** Monitor for signs of severe hypoxemia (low oxygen levels) or hypercapnia (high carbon dioxide levels), such as confusion, cyanosis, or labored breathing.

    - **Ventilator Support:** Provide mechanical ventilation or non-invasive positive pressure ventilation as needed.

    - **Oxygen Therapy:** Administer supplemental oxygen to maintain adequate oxygenation.

    - **Monitoring:** Continuously monitor vital signs, arterial blood gases (ABGs), and response to ventilation.

9. **Bronchitis:**

    - **Assessment:** Monitor for symptoms such as cough, sputum production, and wheezing.

    - **Medications:** Provide bronchodilators and corticosteroids as prescribed.

    - **Supportive Care:** Encourage fluid intake and rest.

    - **Monitoring:** Assess respiratory status and response to medications.

10. Cystic Fibrosis:

- **Assessment:** Monitor for symptoms such as chronic cough, thick sputum, and respiratory infections.
- **Medications:** Administer mucolytics, bronchodilators, and antibiotics as prescribed.
- **Chest Physiotherapy:** Provide or coordinate chest physiotherapy to help clear mucus.
- **Monitoring:** Regularly assess respiratory status, sputum production, and response to treatment.

11. Tuberculosis (TB):

- **Assessment:** Monitor for symptoms such as persistent cough, night sweats, and weight loss.
- **Isolation Precautions:** Implement airborne precautions to prevent transmission.
- **Medications:** Administer anti-tubercular medications as prescribed.
- **Monitoring:** Assess response to treatment and monitor for side effects.

12. Upper Respiratory Infections (e.g., Laryngitis, Sinusitis):

- **Assessment:** Monitor for symptoms such as sore throat, hoarseness, and nasal congestion.
- **Supportive Care:** Provide symptomatic relief with analgesics, decongestants, or saline rinses.
- **Monitoring:** Assess for potential complications or signs of progression.

These conditions require careful monitoring, timely interventions, and coordination with other healthcare professionals to manage acute respiratory issues and support patient recovery.

Urinary System

1. Acute Kidney Injury (AKI):

- **Assessment:** Monitor for signs of decreased urine output, elevated serum creatinine, and electrolyte imbalances.

- **Interventions:**
    - **Fluid Management:** Administer IV fluids to maintain hydration and support kidney function.
    - **Electrolyte Management:** Monitor and correct electrolyte imbalances (e.g., hyperkalemia).
    - **Avoid Nephrotoxins:** Avoid medications or substances that could further impair kidney function.

- **Monitoring:** Regularly assess renal function tests, urine output, and electrolyte levels.

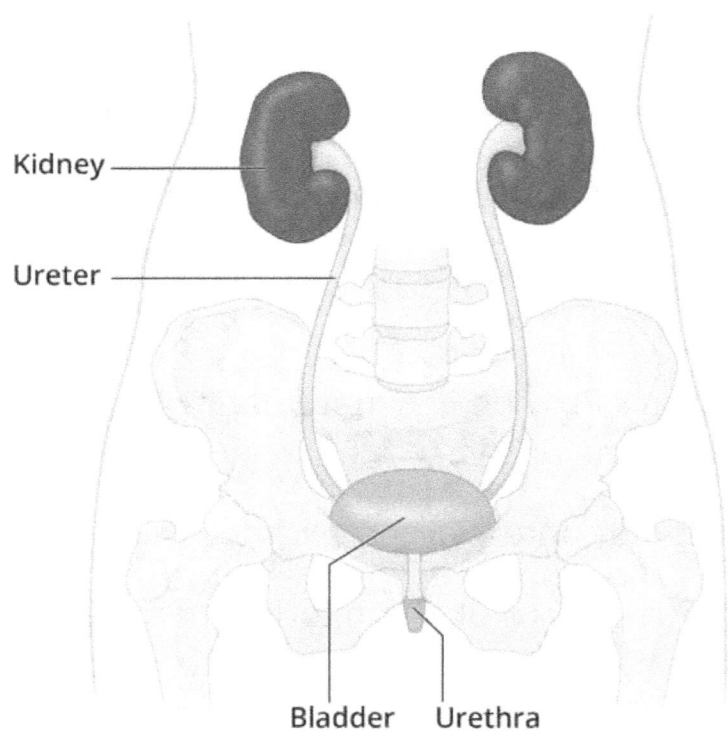

2. Chronic Kidney Disease (CKD) Exacerbation:

- **Assessment:** Monitor for symptoms of fluid overload, elevated blood pressure, and electrolyte imbalances.

- **Interventions:**
    - **Dialysis:** Initiate dialysis if indicated, based on patient's condition and lab results.
    - **Medications:** Manage blood pressure and other complications with appropriate medications.

- **Monitoring:** Regularly check renal function tests, fluid status, and blood pressure.

3. Urinary Tract Infection (UTI):

- **Assessment:** Monitor for symptoms such as dysuria, frequency, urgency, and flank pain.

- **Interventions:**
    - **Antibiotics:** Administer appropriate antibiotics based on culture results.
    - **Hydration:** Encourage fluid intake to help flush the urinary tract.

- **Monitoring:** Regularly assess symptoms and response to antibiotics, and monitor for potential complications such as pyelonephritis.

4. Acute Pyelonephritis:

- **Assessment:** Monitor for symptoms such as fever, flank pain, nausea, and vomiting.

- **Interventions:**

    - **Antibiotics:** Administer IV antibiotics based on culture results.

    - **Hydration:** Provide IV fluids to maintain hydration and support renal function.

- **Monitoring:** Regularly assess vital signs, urine output, and response to treatment.

5. Urolithiasis (Kidney Stones):

- **Assessment:** Monitor for symptoms such as severe flank pain, hematuria, and urinary obstruction.

- **Interventions:**

    - **Pain Management:** Administer analgesics for pain relief.

    - **Hydration:** Encourage fluid intake to help pass the stones and prevent further obstruction.

    - **Surgical Intervention:** Prepare for procedures such as lithotripsy or surgery if indicated.

- **Monitoring:** Regularly assess pain levels, urine output, and signs of obstruction.

6. Urinary Retention:

- **Assessment:** Monitor for symptoms such as inability to void, bladder distension, and discomfort.
- **Interventions:**
  - **Catheterization:** Insert a urinary catheter to relieve acute retention and evaluate bladder function.
  - **Medications:** Administer medications to improve bladder function if appropriate.
- **Monitoring:** Regularly assess bladder distension, urine output, and response to treatment.

7. Bladder Infection (Cystitis):

- **Assessment:** Monitor for symptoms such as dysuria, frequency, urgency, and suprapubic pain.
- **Interventions:**
  - **Antibiotics:** Administer appropriate antibiotics based on culture results.
  - **Pain Management:** Provide analgesics to manage discomfort.
- **Monitoring:** Regularly assess symptoms and response to treatment.

8. Acute Renal Failure:

- **Assessment:** Monitor for symptoms such as oliguria, fluid overload, and elevated blood urea nitrogen (BUN) and creatinine levels.
- **Interventions:**
  - **Dialysis:** Initiate dialysis if needed, based on severity and lab results.
  - **Fluid and Electrolyte Management:** Administer IV fluids and correct electrolyte imbalances.

- **Monitoring:** Regularly check renal function tests, fluid status, and electrolyte levels.

9. Postoperative Urinary Complications:

- **Assessment:** Monitor for complications related to urinary tract surgery, such as urinary leakage or infection.
- **Interventions:**
    - **Catheter Care:** Ensure proper care and monitoring of urinary catheters.
    - **Hydration and Pain Management:** Provide appropriate fluids and manage pain.
- **Monitoring:** Regularly assess for signs of infection, urinary output, and healing.

10. Hematuria:

- **Assessment:** Monitor for blood in the urine, along with any associated symptoms such as pain or urinary obstruction.
- **Interventions:**
    - **Investigation:** Perform diagnostic tests to determine the cause (e.g., imaging studies, cystoscopy).
    - **Supportive Care:** Manage any underlying conditions or complications.
- **Monitoring:** Regularly assess urine color, symptom progression, and response to treatment.

These conditions require timely assessment and intervention to address symptoms, prevent complications, and support patient recovery.

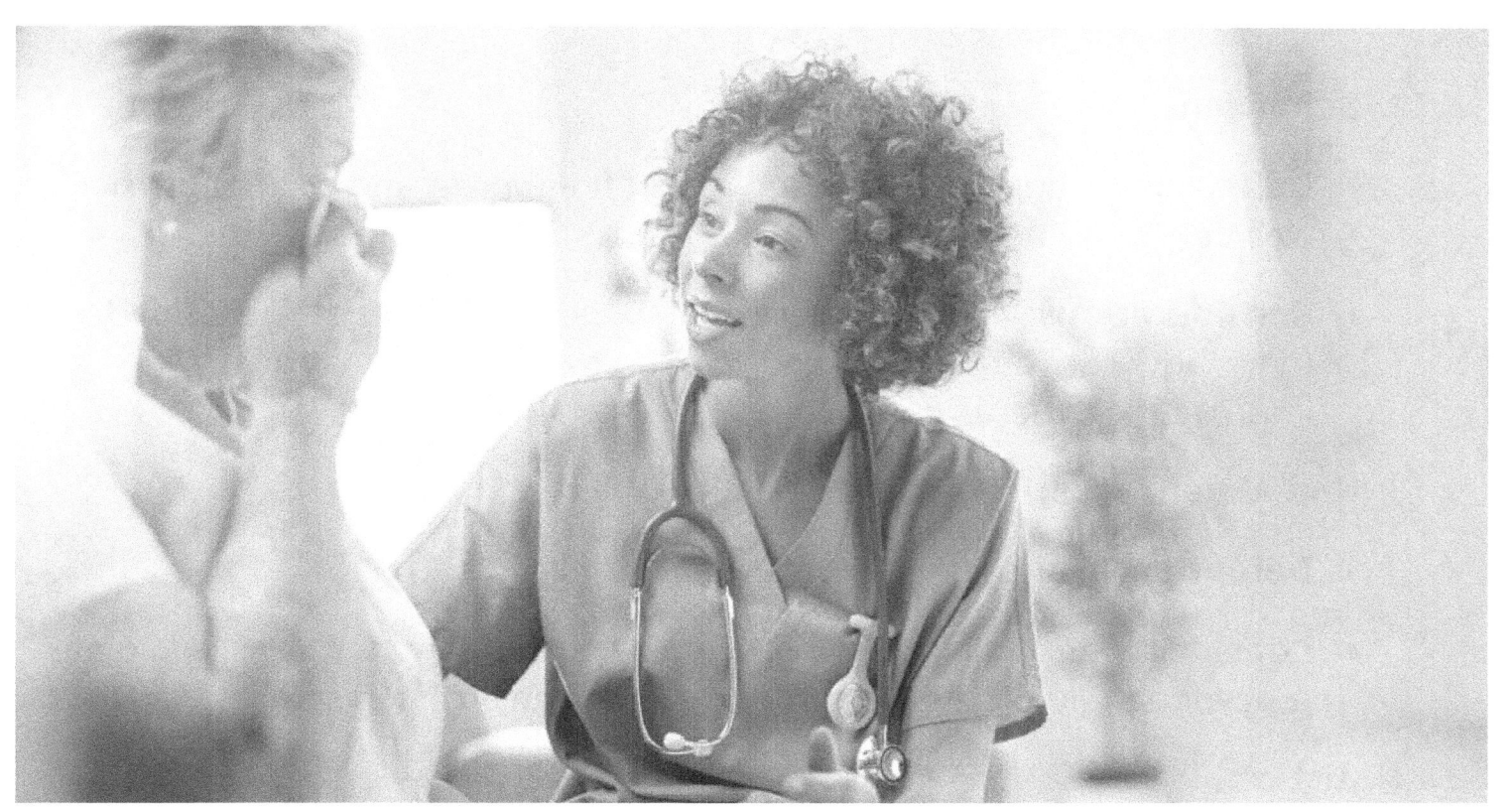

Navigating Patient Care

Ethical Considerations in Patient Care

Ethical considerations in healthcare involve navigating complex issues to ensure that patient care is delivered in a manner that is both morally sound and professionally responsible. Key ethical principles in healthcare include:

1. **Autonomy:**

    - **Definition:** Respecting a patient's right to make their own healthcare decisions.

    - **Considerations:** Ensuring patients are informed about their options, understanding their values and preferences, and obtaining informed consent.

2. **Beneficence:**
   - **Definition:** Acting in the best interest of the patient and promoting their well-being.
   - **Considerations:** Providing care that benefits the patient, considering their physical, emotional, and psychological needs, and striving to improve their overall health.

3. **Non-Maleficence:**
   - **Definition:** Avoiding harm to patients.
   - **Considerations:** Minimizing risks and harm in treatment plans, avoiding procedures with excessive risk, and preventing errors in care.

4. **Justice:**
   - **Definition:** Ensuring fairness and equity in the distribution of healthcare resources.
   - **Considerations:** Providing equal care to all patients regardless of socioeconomic status, race, or other factors, and managing resources fairly.

5. **Confidentiality:**
   - **Definition:** Protecting patient privacy by keeping their health information secure.
   - **Considerations:** Safeguarding patient records, only sharing information with authorized individuals, and adhering to legal and ethical standards regarding privacy.

6. **Veracity:**
   - **Definition:** Being truthful and honest with patients.
   - **Considerations:** Providing accurate information about diagnoses, treatment options, and prognoses, and avoiding deception.

7. **Fidelity:**
   - **Definition:** Honoring commitments and promises made to patients.
   - **Considerations:** Maintaining trust by fulfilling promises, being reliable, and upholding professional obligations.

8. **Informed Consent:**
   - **Definition:** Ensuring that patients understand and agree to the proposed treatment or intervention.
   - **Considerations:** Providing clear and comprehensive information, ensuring patients comprehend their options, and respecting their right to refuse or withdraw consent.

9. **End-of-Life Care:**
   - **Definition:** Addressing ethical issues related to end-of-life decisions.
   - **Considerations:** Discussing advanced directives, palliative care options, and respecting patient wishes regarding life-sustaining treatments.

10. **Professional Boundaries:**
    - **Definition:** Maintaining appropriate relationships with patients.
    - **Considerations:** Avoiding conflicts of interest, maintaining professional conduct, and preventing exploitation or dependency.

11. **Cultural Competence:**
    - **Definition:** Providing care that respects and incorporates patients' cultural values and beliefs.
    - **Considerations:** Understanding cultural differences, avoiding biases, and integrating cultural preferences into care planning.

13. **Resource Allocation:**

    - **Definition:** Making decisions about the distribution of limited healthcare resources.

    - **Considerations:** Balancing individual patient needs with broader societal needs, and making equitable decisions about resource use.

These ethical considerations guide healthcare professionals in making thoughtful, compassionate, and just decisions, ensuring that patient care is delivered with respect, integrity, and professionalism.

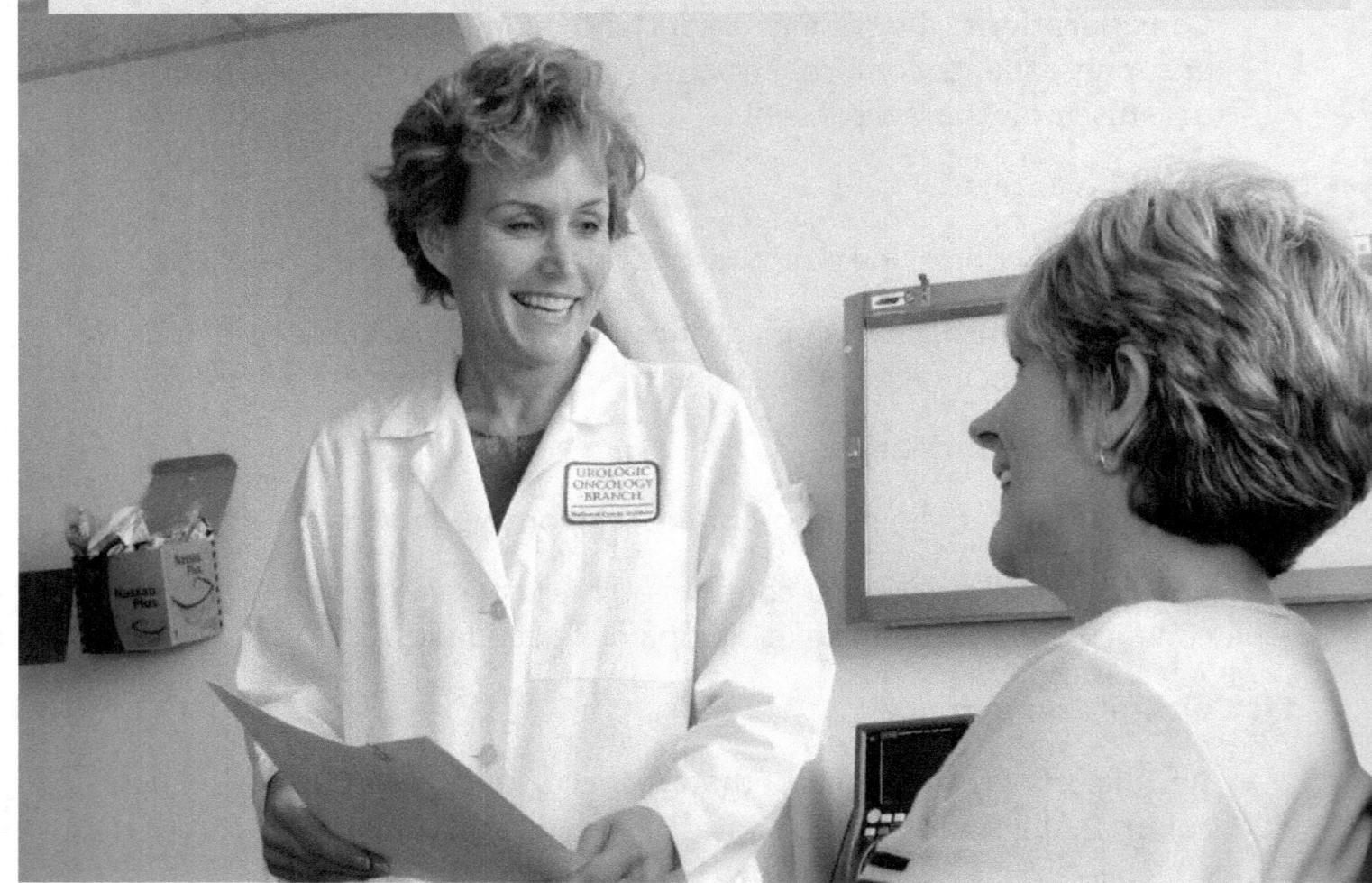

Hospital Nursing Procedures and Protocols

Infection Control and Prevention Measures

Infection control and prevention are critical in healthcare settings to prevent the spread of infections and protect both patients and healthcare workers. Here are key measures:

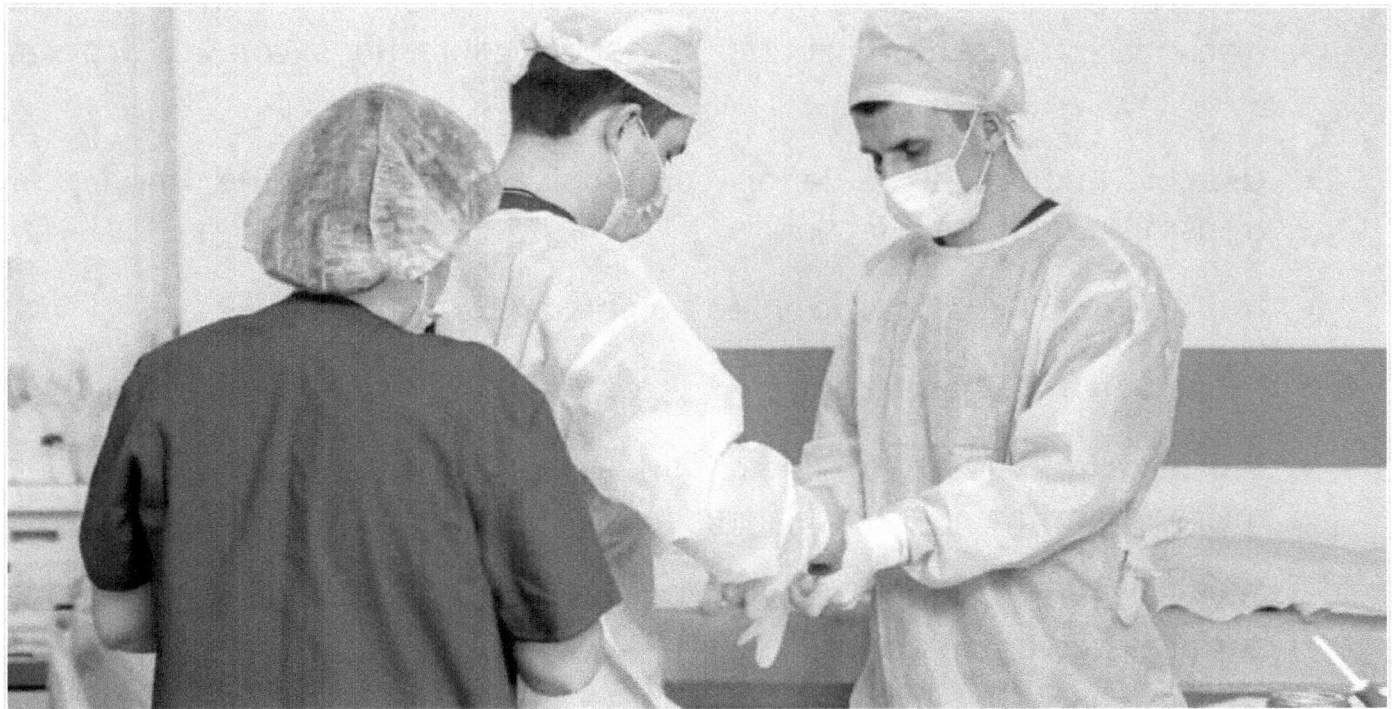

1. **Hand Hygiene:**

    - **Practice:** Wash hands with soap and water or use an alcohol-based hand sanitizer before and after patient contact, after touching potentially contaminated surfaces, and before eating.

    - **Importance:** Reduces the transmission of pathogens.

2. **Personal Protective Equipment (PPE):**
   - **Types:** Gloves, masks, goggles, face shields, gowns.
   - **Usage:** Wear appropriate PPE based on the type of exposure risk (e.g., gloves for contact with bodily fluids, masks for airborne precautions).
   - **Importance:** Protects healthcare workers and prevents the spread of infections.

3. **Isolation Precautions:**
   - **Categories:** Standard precautions (used for all patients) and transmission-based precautions (for specific infections: contact, droplet, airborne).
   - **Usage:** Implement isolation protocols based on the mode of transmission of the infection.
   - **Importance:** Prevents the spread of infectious agents.

4. **Sterilization and Disinfection:**
   - **Sterilization:** Use of heat or chemical methods to kill all microorganisms on medical instruments.
   - **Disinfection:** Use of chemicals to reduce or eliminate pathogens on surfaces and equipment.
   - **Importance:** Ensures that instruments and surfaces are free from infectious agents.

5. **Environmental Cleaning:**
   - **Procedure:** Regularly clean and disinfect surfaces, equipment, and patient areas.
   - **Importance:** Reduces the risk of environmental transmission of infections.

6. **Vaccination:**

    - **Types:** Vaccinations for healthcare workers (e.g., influenza, hepatitis B) and for patients as appropriate.

    - **Importance:** Protects against preventable diseases and reduces the risk of outbreaks.

7. **Safe Injection Practices:**

    - **Procedure:** Use sterile equipment for each injection, and never reuse needles or syringes.

    - **Importance:** Prevents transmission of bloodborne pathogens.

8. **Proper Waste Disposal:**

    - **Types:** Segregate waste into general, biohazardous, and sharp categories.

    - **Procedure:** Dispose of biohazardous and sharp waste in designated containers.

    - **Importance:** Prevents exposure to infectious materials and ensures safe handling.

9. **Respiratory Hygiene and Cough Etiquette:**

    - **Practices:** Encourage patients and staff to cover their mouth and nose with a tissue or elbow when coughing or sneezing, and to dispose of tissues properly.

    - **Importance:** Reduces the spread of respiratory infections.

10. **Patient Care Equipment Management:**

    - **Procedure:** Clean and disinfect reusable equipment after each use, and use single-use items as appropriate.

    - **Importance:** Prevents cross-contamination between patients.

11. **Staff Training and Compliance:**

    - **Training:** Regularly educate healthcare workers on infection control practices and protocols.

    - **Importance:** Ensures adherence to infection control measures and reduces the risk of infection spread.

12. **Surveillance and Monitoring:**

    - **Procedure:** Monitor infection rates and review infection control practices regularly.

    - **Importance:** Identifies trends, evaluates the effectiveness of measures, and guides improvements.

Implementing these infection control and prevention measures helps maintain a safe environment, prevent healthcare-associated infections, and protect the health and safety of patients and staff.

Documentation and Charting Standards

- **Accuracy:** Ensure all entries are precise and reflect the true status of the patient and care provided.

- **Timeliness:** Document information promptly after patient care to ensure details are current and reliable.

- **Completeness:** Include all relevant details, such as patient assessments, interventions, and outcomes, in the chart.

- **Legibility:** Ensure all handwritten entries are clear and legible; use standardized abbreviations and terminology.

- **Confidentiality:** Protect patient privacy by securing records and sharing information only with authorized personnel.

- **Consistency:** Use consistent terminology and formats across all documentation to avoid confusion and ensure clarity.

- **Error Correction:** Correct errors promptly by striking through the incorrect information, initialing the correction, and providing the correct entry.

- **Legal Compliance:** Adhere to legal and regulatory requirements for documentation, including consent forms and compliance with healthcare laws.

- **Professionalism:** Maintain a professional tone and avoid subjective comments; focus on factual, objective information.

These standards help ensure that patient records are accurate, reliable, and useful for ongoing care and legal purposes.

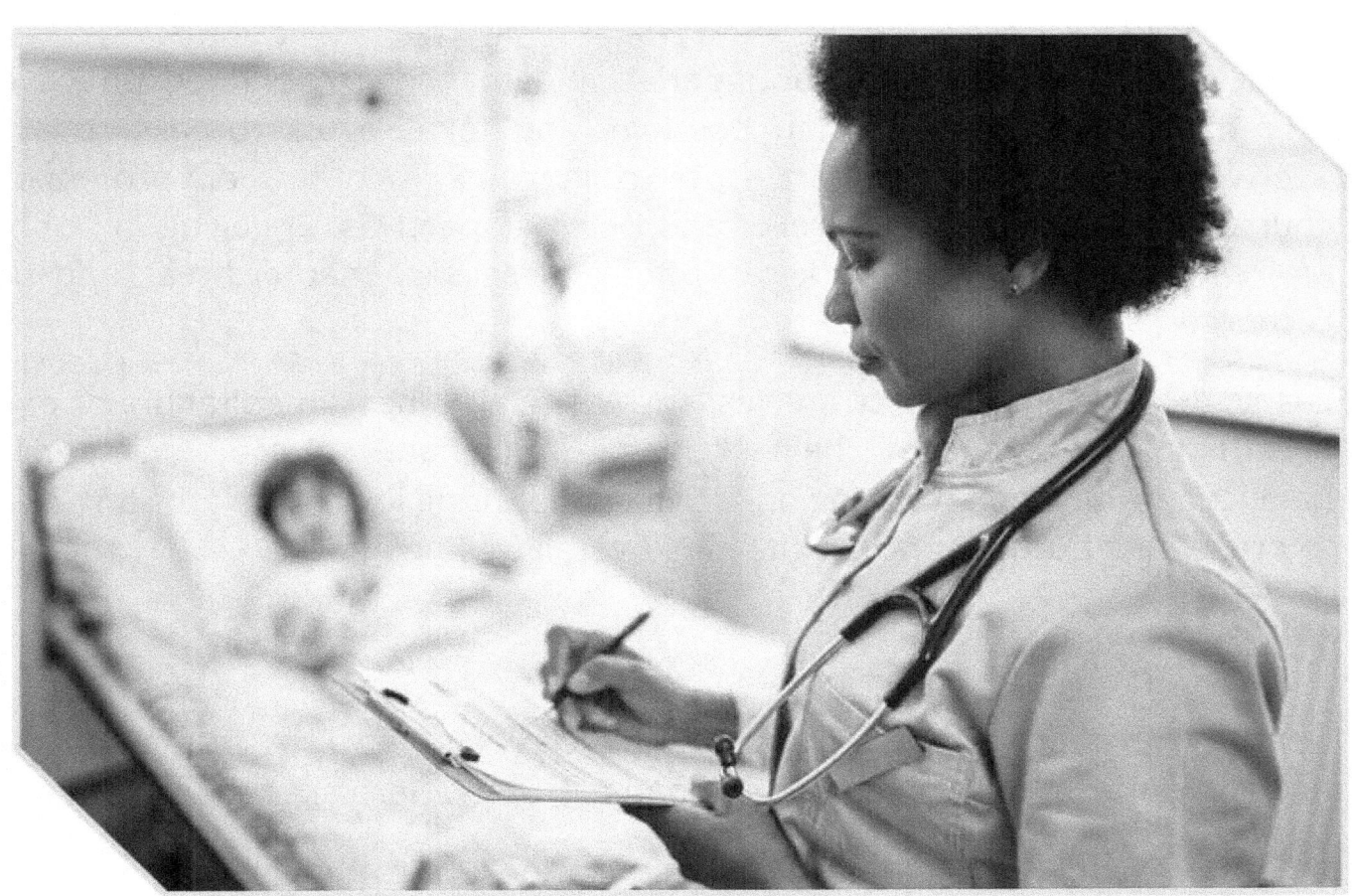

Coping with Challenges in Hospital Nursing

Handling Stress and Burnout

Handling stress and burnout is essential for maintaining personal well-being and professional effectiveness. First, recognizing the signs of stress and burnout—such as fatigue, irritability, and decreased performance—is crucial. Once identified, it's important to take proactive steps to manage these feelings. Regular self-care practices, such as exercise, healthy eating, and sufficient sleep, play a vital role in reducing stress.

Equally important is setting boundaries and managing workload effectively. Prioritize tasks, delegate when possible, and take regular breaks to avoid overworking. Seeking support from colleagues, mentors, or professional counselors can also provide relief and new perspectives. Engaging in hobbies and activities outside of work can offer a necessary mental break and help recharge.

Lastly, developing coping strategies, such as mindfulness, meditation, or deep-breathing exercises, can help manage immediate stressors. Creating a balanced routine and focusing on activities that bring joy and relaxation are key to preventing burnout and maintaining overall well-being.

Dealing with Critical Situations and Emergencies

Dealing with critical situations and emergencies requires a structured approach to ensure effective management and patient safety. Here are key strategies:

1. **Stay Calm and Focused:** Maintain composure to think clearly and make sound decisions. Panic can impair judgment and affect your ability to respond effectively.

2. **Prioritize Actions:** Quickly assess the situation and prioritize tasks based on the severity of the condition. Use the ABCDE approach—Airway, Breathing, Circulation, Disability (neurological status), and Exposure—to identify and address immediate threats.

3. **Communicate Clearly:** Use clear, concise communication to coordinate with team members, provide updates, and delegate tasks. Effective communication ensures that everyone is on the same page and that critical actions are executed promptly.

4. **Follow Protocols:** Adhere to established emergency protocols and guidelines. Familiarize yourself with institutional policies for handling specific emergencies to ensure that you follow best practices. Familiarize yourself with your facilities Code Teams

5. **Utilize Resources:** Access and use available resources, including emergency equipment and specialized personnel, to manage the situation. Ensure that all necessary tools and support are utilized effectively.

6. **Document Thoroughly:** Record all actions taken, observations made, and patient responses. Accurate documentation provides a detailed account of the emergency and is crucial for subsequent care and legal purposes.

7. **Debrief and Reflect:** After the situation is resolved, debrief with your team to discuss what went well and what could be improved. Reflect on the experience to enhance your preparedness for future emergencies.

By staying calm, prioritizing tasks, communicating effectively, and following protocols, you can manage critical situations and emergencies efficiently and ensure the best possible outcomes for patients.

Conclusion

Recap of Essential Points Covered

Accurate patient assessment is the cornerstone of quality care. By performing detailed initial evaluations and continuously monitoring patient conditions, nurses can make informed decisions and adjust care plans as needed. Critical thinking and attention to detail are essential skills for interpreting assessment findings and responding appropriately.

The principles of safe care, including infection control, medication safety, and patient safety, are vital to maintaining a high standard of care. Adhering to infection control protocols, ensuring medication accuracy, and implementing safety measures are all critical practices for preventing complications and protecting patient well-being. Being prepared for emergencies and understanding hospital protocols are also key components of providing effective care.

By integrating these practices, new bedside nurses will be well-equipped to excel in their roles, deliver compassionate and competent care, and contribute positively to patient outcomes and the healthcare team.

Encouragement for Aspiring and Current Nurses

To aspiring and current nurses, remember that your role is both challenging and immensely rewarding. Every day, you have the opportunity to make a profound difference in the lives of your patients and their families. Embrace the journey with resilience and dedication, knowing that your commitment to care and continuous learning will shape the future of healthcare.

Nursing requires a unique blend of compassion, skill, and perseverance. Don't be discouraged by the difficulties you may encounter. Instead, view them as opportunities for growth and development. Lean on your colleagues, seek out mentorship, and stay curious and engaged in advancing your knowledge and skills.

Your ability to connect with patients, provide comfort, and advocate for their needs is invaluable. Celebrate your achievements, no matter how small they may seem, and take pride in the positive impact you have on your patients' lives. Remember that your work is not only about treating illness but also about offering hope, support, and empathy.

Stay passionate about your calling, and never underestimate the difference you make. Your dedication, hard work, and compassion are the foundation of exceptional patient care and contribute to the betterment of the entire healthcare system. Keep pushing forward, stay inspired, and continue to be the beacon of hope and healing that patients and their families need. **You got this!**

Final Thoughts and Resources for Further Learning

As we conclude this eBook, it's important to reflect on the journey of becoming a skilled and compassionate nurse. The knowledge and practices covered here are designed to provide a solid foundation for navigating the complexities of bedside nursing and delivering high-quality patient care. Remember, nursing is a lifelong learning process. Staying current with best practices, evolving technologies, and emerging research is key to maintaining excellence in patient care.

Key Takeaways:

- **Embrace Continuous Learning:** Healthcare is ever-evolving. Commit to ongoing education and professional development to stay ahead and provide the best care possible.

- **Prioritize Self-Care:** Taking care of yourself is crucial for maintaining your well-being and effectiveness as a nurse. Balance your professional responsibilities with personal self-care to prevent burnout.

- **Seek Support and Mentorship:** Don't hesitate to seek guidance from experienced colleagues and mentors. Their insights and support can be invaluable in navigating challenging situations and advancing your career.

Resources for Further Learning:

1. **Professional Organizations:**

   - **American Nurses Association (ANA):** Offers resources, continuing education, and professional development opportunities. ANA Website

   - **National League for Nursing (NLN):** Provides resources for nursing education and professional development. NLN Website

2. **Continuing Education Platforms:**

   - **Medscape:** Offers a variety of free continuing education courses and articles for healthcare professionals. Medscape

   - **Nurse.com:** Provides continuing education courses, webinars, and resources tailored for nurses. Nurse.com

3. **Books and Journals:**

   - **"Fundamentals of Nursing" by Patricia A. Potter:** A comprehensive textbook covering essential nursing concepts and practices.

   - **"Journal of Nursing Scholarship":** Publishes research and reviews on various nursing topics. Wiley Online Library

4. **Online Learning Platforms:**

   - **Coursera:** Offers nursing courses and specializations from top universities. Coursera

   - **Khan Academy:** Provides free educational content that can complement nursing studies. Khan Academy

By leveraging these resources and staying engaged with your professional community, you will continue to grow and excel in your nursing career. Your dedication to learning and improvement is essential to providing exceptional patient care and making a lasting impact in the healthcare field.

Special Formulas

Nursing calculations are essential for ensuring accurate medication administration, fluid management, and patient care. Here are some key formulas and methods commonly used in nursing calculations:

1. Dosage Calculation:

- **Formula:**
$$\text{Dose to Administer} = \left(\frac{\text{Desired Dose}}{\text{Have on Hand}}\right) \times \text{Quantity}$$

- **Example:** If you need to administer 10 mg of a medication, and you have 20 mg tablets on hand, the calculation would be:
$$\text{Dose to Administer} = \left(\frac{10 \text{ mg}}{20 \text{ mg}}\right) \times 1 \text{ tablet} = 0.5 \text{ tablet}$$

2. IV Drip Rate Calculation:

- **Formula:**
$$\text{Drip Rate (gtt/min)} = \left(\frac{\text{Volume to Infuse (mL)}}{\text{Time (min)}}\right) \times \text{Drop Factor (gtt/mL)}$$

- **Example:** If you need to infuse 500 mL of fluid over 4 hours with a drip factor of 20 gtt/mL, the calculation is:
$$\text{Drip Rate} = \left(\frac{500 \text{ mL}}{240 \text{ min}}\right) \times 20 \text{ gtt/mL} \approx 41.7 \text{ gtt/min}$$

3. Flow Rate Calculation (mL/hr):

- **Formula:** $$\text{Flow Rate (mL/hr)} = \frac{\text{Total Volume (mL)}}{\text{Total Time (hr)}}$$

- **Example:** To administer 1,000 mL of fluid over 8 hours, the flow rate is:
$$\text{Flow Rate} = \frac{1000 \text{ mL}}{8 \text{ hr}} = 125 \text{ mL/hr}$$

4. Body Mass Index (BMI):

- **Formula:** $$\text{BMI} = \frac{\text{Weight (kg)}}{\text{Height (m)}^2}$$

- **Example:** For a patient weighing 70 kg and 1.75 meters tall:
$$\text{BMI} = \frac{70}{1.75^2} \approx 22.86$$

5. Medication Concentration Calculation:

- **Formula:** $$\text{Concentration (mg/mL)} = \frac{\text{Total Amount of Drug (mg)}}{\text{Total Volume (mL)}}$$

- **Example:** If a vial contains 500 mg of medication in 250 mL:
$$\text{Concentration} = \frac{500 \text{ mg}}{250 \text{ mL}} = 2 \text{ mg/mL}$$

6. Pediatric Dose Calculation (Based on Weight):

- **Formula:** $$\text{Dose} = \text{Weight (kg)} \times \text{Dosage per kg}$$

- **Example:** For a child weighing 20 kg with a dosage of 5 mg/kg:
$$\text{Dose} = 20 \text{ kg} \times 5 \text{ mg/kg} = 100 \text{ mg}$$

7. Percentage Solutions:

- **Formula:** $\text{Percentage (\%)} = \frac{\text{Amount of Solute (g)}}{\text{Total Solution (mL)}} \times 100$

- **Example:** For a solution with 5 grams of solute in 100 mL: $\text{Percentage} = \frac{5 \text{ g}}{100 \text{ mL}} \times 100 = 5\%$

These formulas are vital for accurate medication administration, fluid management, and patient care, ensuring safe and effective nursing practice.

Burn fluid resuscitation is critical in the management of burn patients to maintain adequate hydration and perfusion. The primary formula used for fluid resuscitation in burn patients is the **Parkland Formula**. Here are the key formulas and concepts:

1. Parkland Formula:

- **Formula:** $\text{Total Fluid Requirement (mL)} = 4 \times \text{Body Weight (kg)} \times \text{Total Body Surface Area (TBSA) burned (\%)}$

- **Example:** For a 70 kg patient with 30% TBSA burns: $\text{Total Fluid Requirement} = 4 \times 70 \text{ kg} \times 30 = 8{,}400 \text{ mL}$

- **Administration:** Half of the calculated volume should be administered in the first 8 hours post-burn, with the remaining half given over the next 16 hours.

2. **Modified Brooke Formula:**

    - **Formula:** Total Fluid Requirement (mL) = 2 × Body Weight (kg) × Total Body Surface Area (TBSA) burned (%)

    - **Example:** For a 70 kg patient with 30% TBSA burns: Total Fluid Requirement = 2 × 70 kg × 30 = 4,200 mL

    - **Administration:** This formula typically does not specify the timing of fluid administration but can be used as a guideline.

3. **Calculating Fluid Resuscitation for Children (e.g., using the Gallons Formula):**

    - **Formula:** Fluid Requirement (mL) = 100 × Body Weight (kg) × Total Body Surface Area (TBSA) burned (%)

    - **Example:** For a 15 kg child with 20% TBSA burns: Fluid Requirement = 100 × 15 kg × 20 = 30,000 mL

4. **Informed Adjustments:**

    - **Hourly Monitoring:** Fluid requirements should be adjusted based on urine output (target of 0.5-1 mL/kg/hr in adults, 1-2 mL/kg/hr in children), vital signs, and clinical status.

    - **Additional Considerations:** Adjustments may be necessary for comorbid conditions, ongoing fluid losses, and changes in patient status.

5. **Electrolyte Management:**
    - **Monitoring:** Ensure proper electrolyte balance by monitoring serum electrolytes and adjusting as needed. Sodium, potassium, and chloride levels should be closely monitored and corrected.

These formulas help guide initial fluid resuscitation but should be tailored based on individual patient needs and ongoing assessments.

Blood, Sweat, and Bedside: The Raw Reality of Bedside Nursing Survival

In an acute care setting, various laboratory tests are used to assess and monitor different body systems. Here's a list of common lab tests organized by body system:

Cardiovascular System

- **Complete Blood Count (CBC)**: Assesses overall health and detects various conditions such as anemia or infection.
- **Basic Metabolic Panel (BMP)**: Measures glucose, calcium, electrolytes, and kidney function.
- **Electrolytes**: Includes sodium, potassium, chloride, and bicarbonate levels.
- **Cardiac Biomarkers**: Includes troponin, BNP (B-type natriuretic peptide), and CK-MB (creatine kinase-MB) for heart injury or heart failure.
- **Lipid Panel**: Measures cholesterol levels (total cholesterol, LDL, HDL, triglycerides).

Respiratory System

- **Arterial Blood Gas (ABG)**: Measures pH, partial pressure of oxygen (PaO2), partial pressure of carbon dioxide (PaCO2), and bicarbonate (HCO3) to assess lung function and acid-base balance.
- **Sputum Culture and Sensitivity**: Identifies bacterial or fungal infections in the respiratory tract.

- **Basic Metabolic Panel (BMP)**: Also includes electrolytes important for respiratory function.

Renal System

- **Renal Function Panel**: Includes tests such as serum creatinine, blood urea nitrogen (BUN), and electrolytes to evaluate kidney function.
- **Urinalysis**: Assesses urine for signs of infection, blood, protein, and other abnormalities.

Hepatic System

- **Liver Function Tests (LFTs)**: Includes tests like AST (aspartate aminotransferase), ALT (alanine aminotransferase), alkaline phosphatase, and bilirubin to evaluate liver function.
- **Ammonia Level**: Can indicate liver dysfunction or hepatic encephalopathy.

Endocrine System

- **Thyroid Function Tests**: Includes TSH (thyroid-stimulating hormone), Free T4 (thyroxine), and Free T3 (triiodothyronine) to assess thyroid function.
- **Blood Glucose**: Monitors blood sugar levels, especially important for patients with diabetes or suspected metabolic disorders.

Hematologic System

- **Complete Blood Count (CBC)**: Evaluates red blood cells, white blood cells, and platelets to assess anemia, infection, and clotting issues.
- **Coagulation Profile**: Includes PT (prothrombin time), aPTT (activated partial thromboplastin time), and INR (International Normalized Ratio) to assess blood clotting.

Gastrointestinal System

- **Basic Metabolic Panel (BMP)**: Includes electrolytes important for gastrointestinal function.
- **Liver Function Tests (LFTs)**: Important for assessing liver health and function.
- **Stool Culture**: Identifies pathogens in cases of gastrointestinal infections.

Musculoskeletal System

- **Serum Calcium and Phosphorus Levels**: Important for bone health and function.
- **Vitamin D Levels**: Assesses vitamin D status, which is crucial for bone health.

These tests help clinicians diagnose, monitor, and manage various acute conditions effectively by providing essential information about the patient's health status.